T0200999

The Agile Approach to Adaptive Research

Wiley Series on Technologies for the Pharmaceutical Industry

Sean Ekins, Series Editor

Computational Toxicology: Risk Assessment for Pharmaceutical and Environmental Chemicals
Edited by Sean Ekins

Pharmaceutical Applications of Raman Spectroscopy
Edited by Slobodan Šašić

Pathway Analysis for Drug Discovery: Computational Infrastructure and Applications
Edited by Anton Yuryev

Drug Efficacy, Safety, and Biologics Discovery: Emerging Technologies and Tools
Edited by Sean Ekins and Jinghai J. Xu

The Engines of Hippocrates: From the Dawn of Medicine to Medical and Pharmaceutical Informatics
Barry Robson and O.K. Baek

Pharmaceutical Data Mining: Approaches and Applications for Drug Discovery
Edited by Konstantin V. Balakin

The Agile Approach to Adaptive Research: Optimizing Efficiency in Clinical Development
Michael J. Rosenberg

The Agile Approach to Adaptive Research

Optimizing Efficiency in Clinical Development

MICHAEL J. ROSENBERG
Health Decisions
Durham, North Carolina

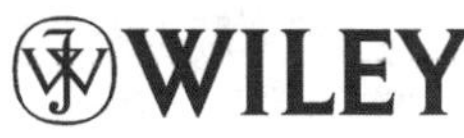

A John Wiley & Sons, Inc., Publication

Published by John Wiley & Sons, Inc., Hoboken, New Jersey.
Published simultaneously in Canada.

Library of Congress Cataloging-in-Publication Data:

Rosenberg, Michael J.
The agile approach to adaptive research : optimizing efficiency in clinical development / Michael J. Rosenberg.
p. ; cm.
Includes bibliographical references and index.
ISBN 978-0-470-24751-8 (cloth)
1. Drug development. 2. Pharmaceutical industry. I. Title.
[DNLM: 1. Drug Discovery—organization & administration. 2. Drug Discovery—methods. 3. Drug Industry—organization & administration. 4. Efficiency, Organizational. QV 744 R813a 2010]
RM301.25.R67 2010
615'.19—dc22 2009040200

Printed in the United States of America.

10 9 8 7 6 5 4 3 2

To Alicia
She knows why.

Contents

Preface

I have seen firsthand how the drug industry developed products that saved many lives and improved the quality of countless others. Novel therapies for heart disease, HIV, and depression are but a few examples. I have the greatest admiration for the many talented people who have enabled the industry to achieve so much for so long. So it is painful to see the industry in the throes of what can only be called a productivity crisis. The cost of producing drugs has risen to prohibitive heights at the same time as the output of new drugs has fallen.

Other long-successful industries have come to face similar challenges; as I write, the automobile industry is the most prominent example. The Big Three automakers that once seemed unassailable fell to unimaginable depths because they could not change with the marketplace:

> *When the price of oil shot up in 1973 and Japanese cars that were better designed, better built, and better looking invaded the American market, the Big Three were caught utterly flat-footed. They have been trying, unsuccessfully, to adapt to the new market conditions ever since—proof that a corporate culture is a very, very hard thing to change.**

The car industry provides a valuable object lesson to the drug industry—an example of what not to do when faced with the need for change. Market conditions are now changing all around the drug industry. The question is whether the industry can change rapidly enough to avoid a period of wrenching decline and move quickly into a new era of invention and prosperity. I believe that the industry can respond. Certainly it has the talent and resources. I have strong convictions about the changes that the industry must make, based on a lifetime of experience in a variety of roles, including extensive direct experience as a physician and clinical researcher.

As a physician, I've worked in rural hospitals in Georgia, some of the world's best known teaching hospitals in Massachusetts, Bangladeshi hospitals with equipment left from British colonial times, and lots in between. In more than 25 years of practicing emergency medicine, I've seen how profoundly new drugs can affect individual lives.

---

* John Steele Gordon, "GM's fall a case of 'creative destruction,'" radio commentary, Marketplace, American Public Media, June 1, 2009.

As a researcher, I've worked on more than 300 clinical programs in a variety of therapeutic and geographic areas. The scope of these programs varied from small first-in-humans studies to large, complex, multinational registration and postmarketing efforts. The budgets have ranged from modest to greater than $100 million.

As an author and a speaker, I've traveled throughout the world, presenting to audiences as small as a handful of people and as large as hundreds. I've offered opinions before high-level panels, physician and policy groups, Congress, and public forums. I have been able to share the experiences of many participants through discussions and one-on-one conversations with physicians, researchers, and consumers.

As a pilot, I learned the value of continuous access to precise, real-time information in exercising control over any complex decision-making process. The contrast between the abundance of timely information that guides decisions in the cockpit and the limited and outdated information available to study and program managers is stark.

As an entrepreneur, I've been able to appreciate the challenges that many corporations face, starting with the minute details required to perform any study, proceeding through the growing pains of startups, and even witnessing the inertia that quickly builds as head count grows. I once wrote the computer code for the programs that processed data; now I have a large staff of specialized, capable individuals who do that. I can focus on keeping the organization as a whole functioning at peak efficiency. Through my company, I have dealt with hundreds of capable industry executives who find themselves enmeshed in well-intentioned corporate procedures that contribute, often indirectly, to frequent delays, cost overruns, and missed opportunities.

My experience convinces me that there is a better way to do clinical research now—not in the future, but now, today. The technology required is available, proven, affordable, and in many cases ubiquitous, having shown its value in other industries faced with similar challenges. When technology provides access to a continuous flow of timely information about the status of the many activities in a clinical study, managers, statisticians, and program coordinators come into their own. They make earlier, smarter decisions, focus resources where they are most beneficial, and produce better results, even if the result is to kill a drug candidate. Ultimately, the flow of information provides the basis for clinical development to proceed much more efficiently, companies to function more effectively, investors to see better returns, and patients to have faster access to new therapies. My own experience shows that using a continuous flow of timely information to manage clinical development gets better results. I recommend this approach because I know that it works.

In this book, I set out to distill my experience into specific, practical steps required to restore the industry's productivity and ensure its prosperity for years to come. My hope is that this book stimulates and challenges you as a reader to help the industry achieve these goals.

MICHAEL J. ROSENBERG

Chapel Hill, North Carolina
October 2009

Acknowledgments

During my career as a researcher and physician, I have enjoyed the good fortune of working with an extraordinarily diverse group of individuals. Some had titles and degrees and instantly recognizable positions of power; some lacked degrees, titles, and recognition by more than a handful of individuals. Some worked in large modern edifices with polished floors, others outdoors with dirt floors. Many spoke English eloquently and were extensively published; others could not read or write, or I could not speak their language. Many lived and worked in the United States and England, while some lived in Bangladesh, rural Brazil, or remote Australia.

However, I spent the greatest part of my professional life with colleagues who occupied neither extreme. In meetings and hallway conversations, over coffee, or during quiet discussions when evening had settled in and most others had left, my colleagues brought new insight and perspective, challenged my ideas, and questioned my logic by every means from a raised eyebrow to boisterous argument. All my colleagues stimulated me to think differently about how an immense, complex, and productive industry works. This book is the product.

Writers know the effort that goes into putting thoughts on paper—the cycle of researching, brainstorming, outlining, drafting, reviewing, revising, and so forth. When much of the material is new, the effort required is even greater. I have been blessed with a superb associate for these tasks, one who embodies the qualities of incisive thinker, candid sounding board, patient researcher, and meticulous editor, Phil Lemmons.

In writing this book, I called on the expertise of many individuals. Those who directly contributed by reviewing sections of the manuscript include Clint Dart, Mark Dibner, Norman Goldfarb, Adam Goldstein, Steve Goodman, Jim Higgins, Susan Levinson, Elliott Levy, Doug Mendenhall, Kelly Murray, Bill Olsen, and Don Powell. I am also indebted to several close friends who provided critical balance between the intensive process of writing and a semblance of real-world perspective: to Peter Mazonson, Nikos Pitsianis, Dale Schneider, and Xiaobai Sun in particular, and many others, my thanks.

I am profoundly grateful for the generous assistance of all these individuals and for the opportunity to learn from each.

M. J. R.

— Chapter 1 —

Opportunity for Efficiency

The fate of large investments and health of many people depend on the results of clinical studies. For one recent trial of a new therapeutic agent for breast cancer, the stakes seemed particularly high. Successful completion of the study would lead to marketing approval for the new agent, bringing women with breast cancer a promising new therapy. The new agent would provide simpler administration and, based on previous work, improve prospects of longer survival. It was the first major product developed by a small biotechnology company. The company's founders were confident that the agent worked well, but the study would stretch their resources to the limit. The company needed both to control expenses and to start generating revenues soon. If the trial succeeded, revenues from the approved product would make the company viable and secure the reputations and livelihoods of the company's principals. If the trial failed, it would destroy the company and derail several careers. The company would have only one chance to get the study right.

In planning discussions for the study, tensions ran as high as the stakes. The small company and the contract research organization (CRO) hired to conduct the study disagreed about how many patients the study required and where to find them. Confirmatory studies of oncology drugs must include detailed assessments of tumor size and progression. Treating and assessing each patient often cost more than $15,000. Furthermore, quickly enrolling enough patients for such studies often presented major challenges. Despite budgets that frequently exceeded $10 million, enrollment delays often caused cost overruns and extended studies beyond planned completion dates. It was hardly surprising that questions about the number of patients required and the best enrollment strategy dominated planning discussions.

Determining the appropriate sample size for clinical studies challenges even the most experienced clinical researchers. For this oncology study, the main determinant of sample size was the size of the treatment effect that the new agent was expected to have on cancer tumors. The greater the treatment effect observed during the trial, the smaller the sample required to provide enough statistical power to demonstrate a difference with the comparator, an existing product representing the standard of care. The smaller the treatment effect, the greater the sample required. However, estimates of treatment effect are at best educated guesses based on limited information.

The principals of the small company believed a strong treatment effect was likely, and thus the study would require relatively few test subjects. The principals were concerned that testing the drug on too many subjects would not only waste scarce resources but also extend the study and delay market entry and revenue generation. Even worse, a larger trial would require the company to raise additional money, imposing substantial delays and a high risk of losing control of the company to outside investors. The company also took an optimistic view of the ability to enroll patients quickly and economically, believing a handful of sites in the United States would be sufficient to meet study timelines for enrollment.

Having seen inadequate sample size undermine other oncology studies, the CRO's statisticians and medical officer focused on the risks of testing the new agent on too few patients. That would prevent the study from producing statistically significant results, wasting the entire effort, and jeopardizing the company's future. The CRO considered a larger sample size based on a more modest estimate of treatment effect prudent. Furthermore, from experience with other oncology studies, the CRO questioned whether the study could enroll enough patients quickly without involving more sites, including some sites in more affordable countries outside the United States.

Despite lengthy discussions, the sponsor and the CRO found it impossible to reach agreement on likely treatment effect, sample size, and enrollment strategy. Both parties considered walking away. The sponsor could easily find another CRO willing to conduct the study with a smaller sample size. The CRO could decline the business to avoid conducting a study doomed from the outset by flawed planning assumptions.

The Adaptive Solution

Instead, the CRO proposed using a technique never before used in a confirmatory study of an oncology product: to wait until midway through the study, look at the actual magnitude of treatment effect observed in enrolled patients, and then use the observed magnitude to recalculate the sample size. Sample-size reestimation (SSRE) is one of the most common techniques in the emerging field of adaptive clinical research. To date, most adaptive techniques allow adjusting a variety of study design elements, such as sample size and ratios for allocating patients to different treatment arms, based on data collected during the study. The principals of the small biotechnology company agreed to the use of sample-size reestimation.

The sponsor also approved an adaptive enrollment strategy based on the CRO's system for real-time monitoring of data on recruitment progress. At inception, the study would use only sites in the United States, but the CRO would arrange for backup sites in Russia to come online rapidly if necessary. Adaptive enrollment belongs to a second class of adaptive techniques aimed not at midcourse optimizations of the study design but at optimizing key study operations based on performance metrics continuously derived from study data. Operational adaptations can adjust enrollment strategy, the approach to monitoring study sites, allocation of key resources, and many other aspects of study operations.

The CRO launched the study based on a larger, more conservative sample size, with provision for adjustment based on actual trial data when enrollment reached half the expected number of patients. Real-time data on recruitment progress soon showed the need to activate the backup sites in Russia. The additional sites quickly accelerated enrollment, hastening the date of sample-size reestimation. At the halfway point, study managers declared an interim database lock (restricting write access to the database preparatory to analysis). Techniques for rapid data validation and analysis enabled completing the interim lock in a single day. That same afternoon, analysis of actual study data showed that the treatment effect fell between the initial conservative estimate and the more optimistic estimate by the sponsor.

The good news was that a 25% reduction in sample size would allow meeting statistical goals and saving more than $1,000,000 in direct costs. The bad news was that completing the remainder of the study in typical fashion would still cost more than the sponsor had hoped. The CRO recommended the use of adaptive monitoring for the balance of the study. Instead of sending monitors to visit all remote sites the same number of times at the same intervals throughout the study, study managers would allocate site visits based on need, as indicated by metrics on site performance, such as query rate, the number of queries outstanding, and the mean time to resolve queries at each site. Monitors would also use an electronic tool to facilitate their work on site. Without compromising data quality, adaptive allocation of site visits and advanced monitoring tools reduced the need for expensive monitoring personnel, the amount of travel required, and overall monitoring expenses.

In the end, three key adaptive elements—sample-size reestimation, adaptive enrollment, and adaptive monitoring—allowed completing the study within the sponsor's budget and a year ahead of schedule. Shortening the study and reducing sample size saved a relatively modest $1.9 million in direct expenses. The indirect benefits were much greater. The breast-cancer treatment was the first in its category to reach the market. It had sales of $329 million in the first year. Reaching the market earlier allowed an additional year to market the product with patent exclusivity and, over time, generated an additional $299 million in profit. Best of all, the new therapeutic agent is helping improve the treatment of women with breast cancer today.

This story about one small biotech and its CRO may point to a better future for an industry that has struggled to develop new drugs in recent years despite vast R&D expenditures. The disappointing output of new drugs leaves no doubt about the need for greater efficiency in clinical research. This book explains an approach that uses information and communications technologies together with methodological improvements to make clinical development much more efficient. These changes can help shape a brighter future for the pharmaceutical industry.

An Industrial Success Story

For decades, the pharmaceutical industry has enjoyed numerous and impressive successes, both scientific and financial. Among the most spectacular examples, HmG co-A reductase inhibitors ("statins") have contributed to a dramatic reduction in deaths from atherosclerotic heart disease, long a leading cause of mortality in western nations.[1] More than 300 drugs are now available for the treatment of rare diseases (defined as those that affect fewer than 200,000 people in the United States); fewer than 10 such drugs existed before the 1983 approval of the Orphan Drug Act.[2] Drugs such as insulin sensitizers have allowed improving glucose levels for people with type 2 diabetes, bringing hope to approximately 160 million individuals worldwide.[3] HIV was a uniformly fatal disease only a decade ago, but an individual diagnosed with the infection today has a life expectancy approaching that of the general population.[4] A new generation of anticoagulants greatly reduces thromboembolic complications of orthopedic surgery and thus reduces the risk of myocardial infarction.[5]

Providing such compelling health benefits has brought the drug industry substantial rewards. For example, Pfizer's Lipitor (atorvastatin, the leading statin drug) generated sales of $83.5 billion from its introduction in 1997 through 2007. Lipitor sales for 2006 and 2007 were $12.9 billion and $12.7 billion, respectively.[6,7]

Signs of Trouble Ahead

Despite such striking medical and financial successes, the pharmaceutical industry today faces a deepening crisis: inefficiency in its core business, the development of new drugs. Impressive increases in research-and-development (R&D) spending have failed to produce corresponding increases in the output of drugs that are truly new, that is, not reformulations or combinations of existing drugs. Industry investments in R&D totaled $214.3 billion just in the period from 2004 to 2007, culminating in a record expenditure of $58.8 billion in 2007, including expenditures by biotechnology companies.[8] However, according to one analysis, although the industry has doubled its annual investment in R&D over the past decade, output of new drugs has fallen 60%.[9] This is consistent with a decline in approved new drugs from 53 in 1996 to 23 in 2007, a drop that occurred while members of the Pharmaceutical Research and Manufacturers of America (PhRMA) increased R&D expenditures from $16.9 billion annually to $44.5 billion (Figure 1-1).

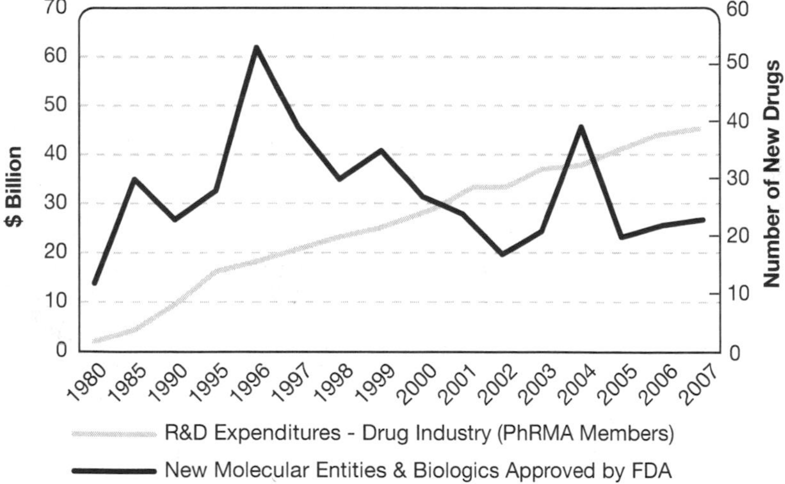

Figure 1-1. Expenditures to develop new drugs and biologics have surged in recent years to unprecedented levels but failed to increase output of approved novel products, that is, new drugs and biologics excluding reformulations and combinations of existing products.

Source: Pharmaceutical Research and Manufacturers of America, Food and Drug Administration Center for Drug Evaluation and Research.[10]

Critics charge the drug industry with exaggerating its R&D expenditures. They object to including indirect considerations such as potential gains from alternative investments.[11,12] However, many businesses consider such factors when making investment decisions. Furthermore, those estimating R&D costs argue that it is appropriate to assign a monetary value to time costs when any return comes only after lengthy periods of investment.[13] Since the drug industry's out-of-pocket R&D expenditures have also increased significantly, there is no denying the general point: R&D expenditures have increased without a corresponding increase in the output of new drugs.

Converging Challenges

About 80% of the drugs that enter clinical trials never emerge and thus generate no revenues to offset development costs.[14] Furthermore, the current round of development casualties comes as the industry faces an unprecedented series of business challenges, including:

- a proliferation of cost controls such as the formularies of private and public health insurers, which limit access to expensive new drugs;
- the rise of generic alternatives to brand-name products;
- a wave of patent expirations on an aging generation of highly profitable "blockbuster" drugs that sustain the industry's business model;
- the Food and Drug Administration's (FDA's) delaying or withholding approvals and requiring stronger warning labels following recalls of major medications such as Vioxx (rofecoxib).

Lipitor again illustrates. Pfizer reaped a bonanza from this blockbuster. Indeed, Warner Lambert's ownership of Lipitor inspired Pfizer's hostile acquisition of the company for more than $90 billion in 2000.[15] However, Lipitor's patent exclusivity begins to expire in 2010.* Pfizer was counting on its own promising candidate in the same therapeutic class, torcetrapib, to replace the revenues soon to be lost to generic versions of Lipitor and other statins. Pfizer's disappointing trials of torcetrapib had severe yet typical repercussions. After investing almost $1 billion, Pfizer abandoned the drug in December 2006 without filing for regulatory approval.[16] The announcement slashed Pfizer's market value by $21.3 billion in a single day,[17] precipitated layoffs, and underscored the risks of relying on a handful of blockbuster drugs. Pfizer litigated to delay the introduction of Indian manufacturer Ranbaxy Laboratories' generic version of Lipitor before Ranbaxy agreed to a 20-month delay in many markets.[18] Pfizer's January 2009 agreement to purchase Wyeth for $68 billion seems at least in part a response

* The first of a series of patents expires in March 2010, but because of ongoing litigation and other patents, precisely when market exclusivity in the United States will be lost remains unclear, and market exclusivity varies in different parts of the world. Most bets are that June 2011 will be the critical date. However, if Pfizer's recent deal with Ranbaxy stands, it puts that date in doubt in the United States.

to expected declines in sales of Lipitor and other drugs with expiring patents.[19] Such maneuvers by Pfizer and other drug companies protect and extend exclusive market positions. However, expensive acquisitions are a poor substitute for the development and introduction of compelling new products. Mergers and acquisitions do not make a long-term strategy.

Disappointing trials hurt small companies even more than industry giants. Table 1-1 shows the harsh consequences of having a lead product fail in clinical testing.

Table 1-1. The effect of failed clinical testing of lead products on share prices of small companies.

Company	Lead Candidate	Indication	Share Price Effect
Renovis	NXY-059	Stroke	–76%
Nuvelo	Alfimeprase	Arterial obstruction	–79%
Telik	Telcyta	Lung, ovarian cancer	–71%
Dynavax	Tolamba	Ragweed allergy	–30%
Threshold	Glufosfamide	Pancreatic cancer	–57%

Source: San Francisco Chronicle, Mar. 11, 2007.[20]

Like Pfizer, much of the drug industry clings to the blockbuster model despite growing evidence against its validity. Driven by cost concerns, especially as expressed through formulary preferences, sales of generics have flourished. In 2007, generics accounted for two-thirds of prescriptions written in the United States (Figure 1-2).

Many formularies already favor simvastatin, a generic version of Zocor, Merck's blockbuster statin. Simvastatin came off patent in 2006.[22] Zocor's acceptance in formularies plunged after the introduction of a generic version. This foreshadows Lipitor's fate.

The Struggle to Replace Lost Revenues

In recent years, the drug industry has had far too many torcetrapibs and too few new Lipitors to sustain its current business model. Between 2007 and 2011, patents will expire on 14 major drugs, resulting in estimated losses of $100 billion in sales of brand-name drugs to generic competitors.[23] No industry could easily replace such a huge loss of revenue. A recent analysis of 14 leading drug companies identifies corresponding peer groups of old drugs rolling off patent and new drugs coming on the market. A compari-

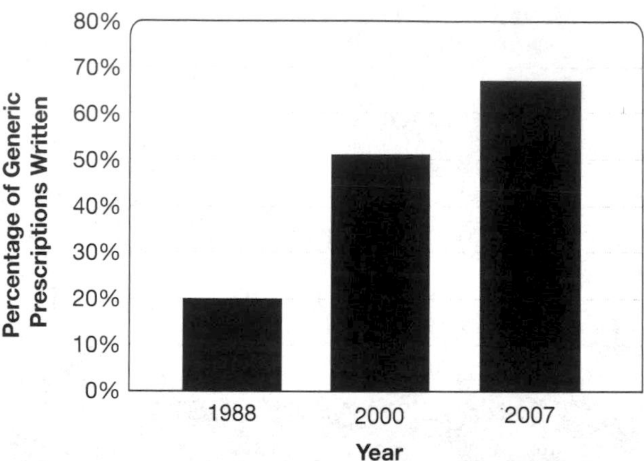

Figure 1-2. Prescriptions for generic drugs represented 67% of all prescriptions in the United States in 2007.

Source: The New York Times.[21]

son of expected revenues lost by the group of old drugs and gained by the new ones concludes that in 2007, the 14 firms generated only $0.77 for each $1.00 of lost sales. The worst is yet to come. The analysis projects a decline by 2012 to only $0.23 in new revenue to replace each $1.00 lost.[24] A 2006 report indicated Pfizer executives referred to the looming expiration of patents on five major drugs in a five-year period as "the cliff."[25] Patent cliff has become part of the industry's vocabulary.

The combination of rising generic sales, aging blockbusters, high development costs, and low success rates has taken a toll on the market capitalization of most large drug companies (Figure 1-3). Abbott was the only company whose market capitalization did not drop substantially between December 30, 2000 and June 30, 2008. It is probably not a coincidence that Abbott derives less than half of its revenues from pharmaceuticals. In another comparison over roughly the same period (December 2000 to February 2008), the stocks of 15 major drug companies lost $850 billion in value.[26]

Growth of the drug industry's global profits has been slowing for almost a decade despite spectacular successes in the same period. Blockbusters like Lipitor, Plavix (clopidogrel), Advair (salmeterol/fluticasone), and Viagra (sildenafil) were not enough to reverse the trend. Between 2000 and 2007, the annual growth rate in global sales fell by almost one-half (Figure 1-4).

Although a declining growth rate raises concerns, a decline in revenues indicates a serious problem for any industry. IMS Health forecasts declining U.S. revenues for the drug industry in 2009. The industry has not experienced such a contraction for more than a half century. Murray Aitken,

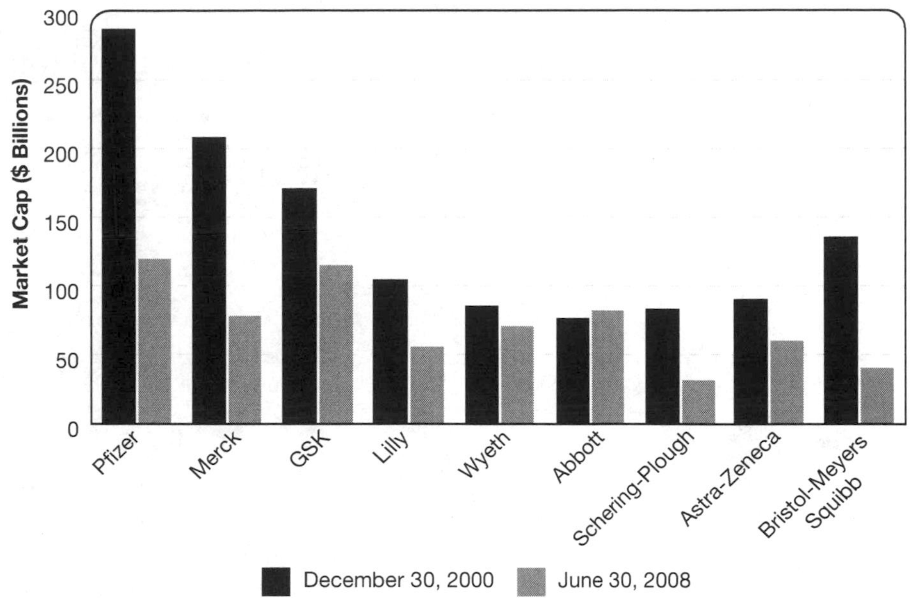

Figure 1-3. Almost all of the leading companies in the pharmaceutical industry saw their market capitalization decline substantially between December 30, 2000 and June 30, 2008, before the sharp across-the-board decline in financial markets in late 2008.

Source: CottonMoehrke Financial Group UBS; Wolfram Alpha LLC.

senior vice president of IMS Health, highlighted lack of innovation as an underlying issue. "It's much more difficult now if you are not a very innovative product with a very strong clinical profile to be launching into a therapy area where leading generics are available, and expect to get a first-line position," Aitken said.[28]

The decline in revenues is but the latest sign that the drug industry should treat the disparity between R&D spending and output of compelling new products as an urgent problem. Certainly pharmaceutical development is expensive and inherently risky. Failure can happen anywhere on the long road from discovery through preclinical development, clinical testing, regulatory submission, and approval. Developing a new drug takes 10–15 years, failure is the norm, and the accumulating costs stagger the imagination. Four recent estimates of per-drug development costs are $802 million,[14] $868 million,[29] $882 million,[30] and $1.65 billion.[31] Although these figures include a variety of indirect costs, the out-of-pocket investments are themselves enormous, especially for clinical development (see below).

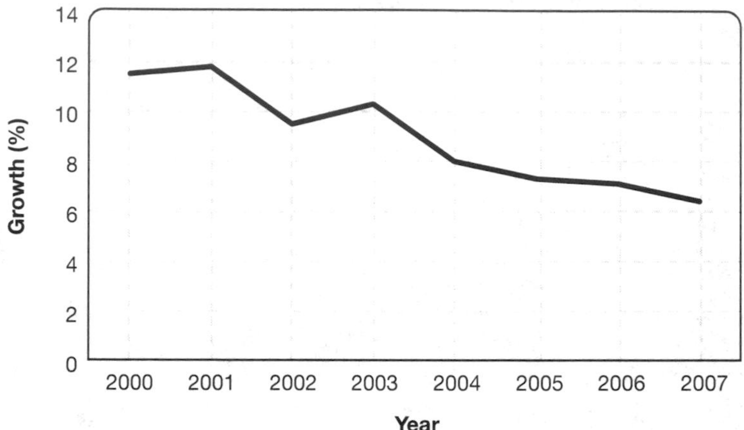

Figure 1-4. Global sales growth over previous year for pharmaceuticals. Between 2000 and 2007, the total world market grew from $365 to $712 billion, but the rate of growth fell by almost one-half.

Source: IMS Health Market Prognosis, Mar. 28, 2008.[27]

Clinical Research Is the Key

Both costs and risks are greatest in the clinical stage of development. Most new drugs fail in clinical testing. Clinical studies also consume the bulk of the drug industry's out-of-pocket, per-drug R&D expenditures and development time. Clinical research accounts for 70% of the $403 million in average out-of-pocket costs and 64% of average development time of 11.8 years[14] (Figure 1-5).

Furthermore, the proportion of out-of-pocket R&D expenditures devoted to clinical studies is growing. Annual growth rates for out-of-pocket clinical R&D costs were 6.1% for approvals in the 1970s and 1980s and almost twice as great, 11.8%, for approvals in the 1980s and 1990s. Out-of-pocket preclinical costs declined from 7.8% to 2.3% on drugs approved in the corresponding periods.[14]

Thus, if the drug industry is to reduce the investment and time required to develop new drugs, clinical development demands scrutiny. There are two major ways to save on clinical development. The first is to conduct successful studies faster and in the process bring drugs to market at lower cost. The second, equally important given the high failure rate, is to find ways to identify drug failures earlier, before large, long, and expensive phase II and phase III trials. These trials consume most of the time devoted to clinical development, whether the therapeutic agent is a biologic or a more traditional compound[32] (Figure 1-6). This makes a powerful economic argu-

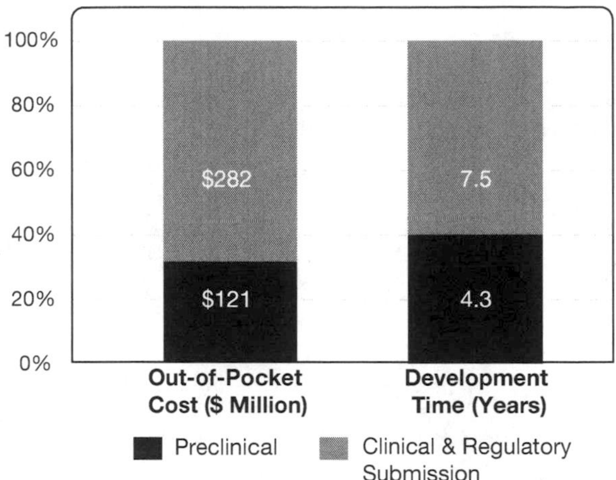

Figure 1-5. Clinical trials and submissions for regulatory approval account for an average of 70% of the direct costs of drug development and 64% of development time.

Source: DiMasi et al. 2003.[14]

ment for research methodologies that allow learning more about new drugs earlier in the development process. Every R&D budget should address the search for new methodologies as well as new drugs.

The comparable time required to develop biotech drugs—many from aggressive startup companies—suggests that pharma giants do not have a monopoly on inefficient development practices. The problem extends across different types of companies, therapeutic agents, and treatment classes. The time required to win approval does vary by therapeutic area. Oncology and neurological drugs (such as antidepressants and Alzheimer's treatments) are most complex and take longest. Anti-infectives and gastrointestinal (GI)/metabolic drugs typically gain approval fastest. However, all therapeutic areas are experiencing longer timelines and disappointing approval rates.

Behind the High Costs of Clinical Development

Drug development has become considerably more complex in recent years. There are more studies, more subjects and procedures per study, and more restrictive criteria for entry into studies. Drug discovery is benefiting from the explosion of knowledge and technology associated with the genetics revolution, computational chemistry, and high-throughput screening. Preclinical timelines have decreased. However, longer clinical phases have offset preclinical gains, increasing overall development times.

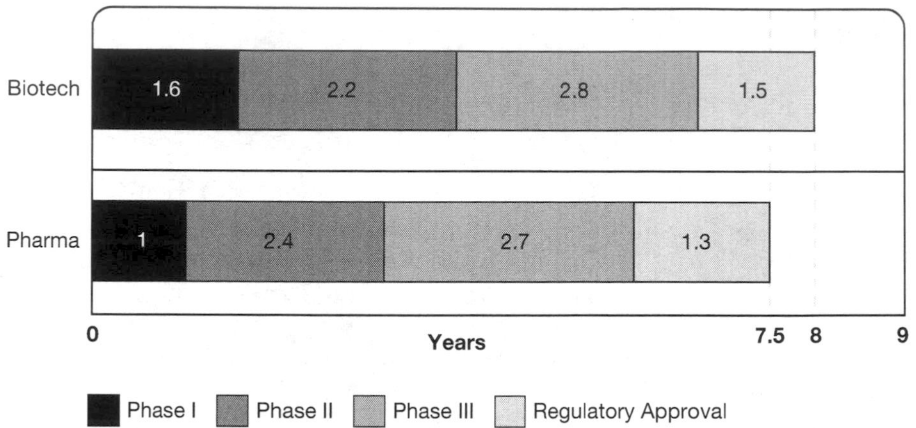

Figure 1-6. Expensive phase II and phase III clinical trials account for most of the time in clinical development.

Source: DiMasi and Grabowski 2007.[32]

The growing size of clinical studies is a major contributor to growing costs. For example, the number of subjects involved in clinical testing for each submission to the FDA for approval of a new drug grew 562% between 1977–80 and 1998–2001, from 1,576 to 5,621[33] (Figure 1-7).

Increases in the number of inclusion criteria and the number of procedures required for each subject have also increased costs. The Tufts Center for the Study of Drug Development reports that the number of inclusion criteria for each study more than doubled between the 1999–2002 and 2003–2006 periods.[34] The same Tufts researchers obtained information from DataEdge showing large percentage increases in the number of medical procedures administered to each patient in phase I, phase II, and phase III trials from 1990 to 1997 (Figure 1-8). The largest increase, 120%, was in the number of procedures in large, expensive phase III trials.

Study protocols continued the trend of requiring increasing numbers of procedures between 1999 and 2005. The number of unique procedures across all therapeutic areas grew at an annual rate of 6.5%. In 2005, the median number of unique procedures per protocol in trials across all phases and therapeutic areas reached 35. The frequency of performing procedures grew even more rapidly, at an average annual rate of 8.7%.[35]

High Costs and Increasing Prices

In sum, the complexity, magnitude, and cost of clinical testing have increased steadily in recent decades, driving R&D expenditures to new heights. The drug industry has maintained some growth in profits, but the

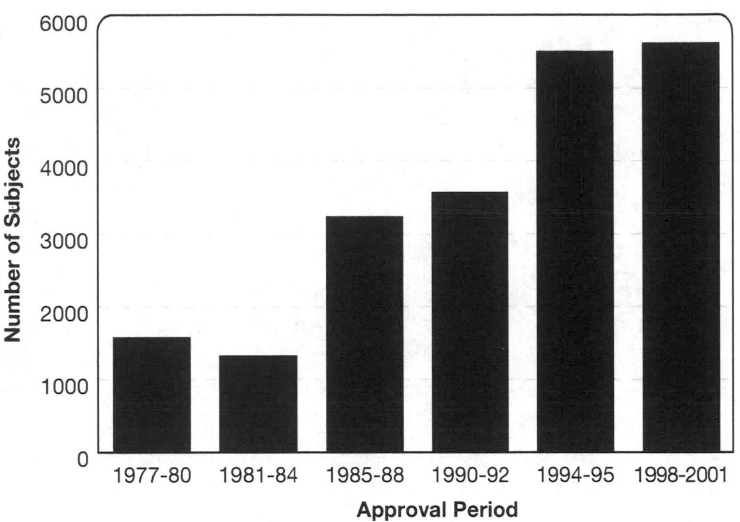

Figure 1-7. Mean number of test subjects in clinical trials for new drugs (new molecular entities or NMEs) by specified periods. The number of test subjects increased by a factor of 4 from the period 1981–1984 to the period 1998–2001.

Source: Boston Consulting Group, 1993; Peck, Food and Drug Law J, 1997; Parexel, 2002.[33]

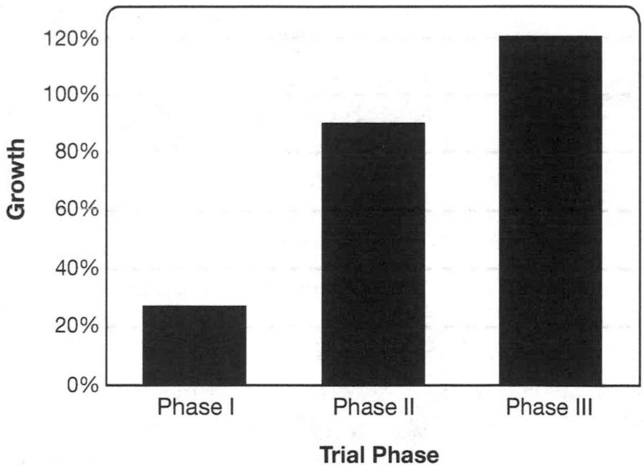

Figure 1-8. The number of medical procedures administered to each patient in clinical trials increased by large percentages from 1990 to 1997, especially in larger phase II and phase III trials.

Source: DiMasi et al. 2003.[14]

strain is evident. For example, pharmaceuticals have taken a larger and larger percentage of national health-care expenditures in the United States. During the decade of the 1990s, the average annual percentage increase in national expenditures for prescription drugs was 12%. That is double the increase in the same period for physician and clinical services and more than double the increase for hospital care. The annual expenditures are still increasing. However, the rate of increase declined from 15% in 2000 to 11% in 2003 and 6% in 2005[36] (Figure 1-9).

Prices for prescription drugs increased from $28.67 to $68.26 from 1994 to 2006, an average of 7.5% per year, approximately triple the annual rate of inflation. The average branded prescription price was higher still: $111.02 in 2006. It is a reasonable inference that the drug industry has increased prices at such a rate at least in part to maintain some growth in profits. The rate of growth in profits has declined anyway. Although the industry argues that the treatments it provides remain less costly than surgical alternatives in some therapeutic areas, the trends in pricing and profitability speak for themselves. Presumably, the industry would rejoice if it could maintain growth in profits while moderating price increases. Reducing development costs and bringing greater numbers of new drugs to market would make this possible. Revenues would grow from additional sales of new products. The strategy of growth through price increases has given the industry a new set of problems (see below, "Cost of Inefficiency: Public Backlash").

The prices of some innovative new oncology drugs have provoked extreme reactions. Patients believe their survival may depend on gaining access to the new treatments but costs are prohibitive. Erbitux (cetuximab), first used as a treatment for colon cancer, costs $17,000 per month. Zevalin (ibritumomab), used to treat some rare forms of lymphoma, costs $24,000 per month. Avastin (bevacizumab) costs $4,400 per month.[38] A 2004 *New England Journal of Medicine* editorial noted that FDA approval of Avastin alone could add $1.5 billion a year to the nation's health costs.[39] *The New York Times* reported in July 2008 that the price of Avastin has increased to almost $100,000 per patient per year, generating sales of $3.5 billion globally, including $2.5 billion in the United States. Yet the same article reports the drug prolongs life by only a few months, and recent research has called even this benefit into question.[40] The industry has indicated on many occasions that high development costs mandate such high prices for novel therapies. Nevertheless, high prices reveal the strain of high development costs.

The industry appears committed to substantial price increases as a strategy for growth despite hard economic times and widespread concerns about already unsustainable health-care costs. In April 2009, the industry increased prices on some drugs, including treatments for leukemia and erectile dys-

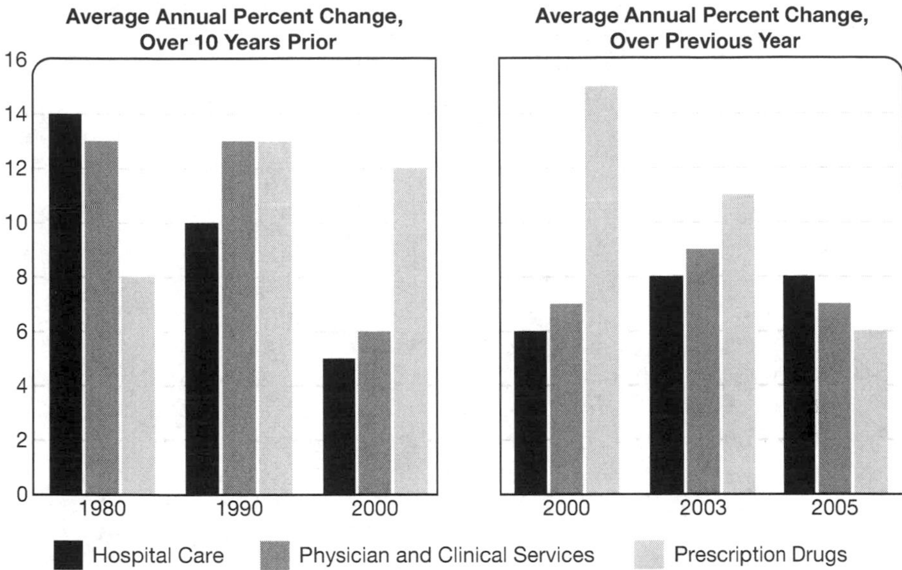

Figure 1-9. The drug industry has consumed an increasing percentage of national health-care expenditures, in part because of increases in prescription drug prices.
Source: Kaiser Family Foundation, Oct. 2004.[37]

function, by more than 20%. Rates on other drugs increased by about 10%.[41] The Consumer Price Index decreased 0.4% for the 12 months ending in March 2009, the first 12-month decline in more than half a century.[42]

Cost of Inefficiency: Public Backlash

Aggressive price increases exact a cost in the goodwill of patients, health-care providers, and policymakers. Whether high drug prices fairly reflect actual development costs is debatable. However, there is no debate about how cancer patients react to such prices. When the monthly cost of some drugs can exceed the patient's annual income, many cancer patients believe they face the highwayman's ultimatum: your money or your life. The resulting outcries may exacerbate a backlash against the drug industry that is all too evident in public opinion surveys. Half of the U.S. public holds an unfavorable opinion of the industry, and one-quarter has a "not at all favorable" opinion.[43]

Indeed, the public now ranks the drug industry with the pariahs of the business world. Like Big Oil, the drug industry ranks a little higher in public esteem than Big Tobacco. This result is startling for an industry in the business of providing treatments for human disease and suffering. How is it possible for an industry with this benign mission to earn public disdain comparable to that of industries that sell lethal and addictive products or an essential and diminishing natural resource? Many people can remember a time when much of the public viewed the drug industry very differently. Today's corporate villain was once a modern miracle worker providing new classes of drugs with indisputable value, such as antibiotics and antidepressants.

The drug industry cannot dismiss measures of the public's disapproval as a reflection on the health-care system as a whole rather than the drug industry specifically. Surveys show the drug industry ranking below every other part of the health-care system in public esteem. For example, hospitals have a 78% favorable rating, of which 39% is very favorable. Physicians score even higher favorability ratings. In stark contrast, only 9% of Americans think pharmaceutical companies are "generally honest and trustworthy." No less than 69% of the American public considers high profits made by drug companies a very important factor in causing higher health costs.[37] The industry strategy of explaining high prices by simultaneously pointing to high development costs and running consumer advertising campaigns has not played well with the people who consume the products and the entities that foot the bill.

"Rightly or wrongly, drug companies are now the number one villain in the public's eye when it comes to rising health-care costs," according to Kaiser Family Foundation President Drew E. Altman. "People want to rein in the cost of prescription drugs, and just about anything we poll on with that aim gets public support."[44]

Growing Pressures Mandate Greater Efficiency

Public opinion is not the only source of intensifying pressure on the drug industry to reduce development costs. Other noteworthy pressures include the trend toward segmenting populations by markers that predict response (genetics and proteins and metabolites), the sense that research has long since identified most potential "blockbusters," and growing competition from more nimble biotechnology companies and low-cost drug companies in emerging countries.

The Effect of Genetically Targeted Medicines

Despite its unquestioned benefits, the genetics revolution and its offshoots increase pressure for more efficient drug development. There are several reasons. First, with current methods, developing products such as recombinant proteins is even more costly than developing a conventional chemical compound. Developing a typical new biologic costs $1.2 billion.[32] Recovering such high development costs presents an enormous challenge. One of the great scientific and medical by-products of the genetics revolution—the possibility of practicing individualized medicine based on the distinct genetic makeup of each patient—provides exciting benefits, such as increasing the odds of successful treatment and reducing the likelihood of side effects. However, the same genetic targeting also restricts the market for each product to patients with the appropriate genetic profile.

A recent analysis examines the likely effects on development strategy and market economics of the complex interplay between the benefits of such targeted medicines and potential economic drawbacks such as smaller market size. On scenarios characterized as "sustained future" and "bright future," projected lifetime gross profit for such medicines declines from approximately $4 billion today to estimated figures of $2.15 billion and $2.4 billion. The analysis takes an optimistic view on the ability to charge very high prices for such medicines. It concludes: "Stratified medicine changes the incentives for innovation, alters the drug and diagnostic development process, complicates regulatory review, and further extends the fragile reimbursement structure. But if all players adapt, patients will reap the benefits of better clinical outcomes, payers will spend less on ineffective treatments, and manufacturers will remain economically viable and continue to develop new products."[45]

Despite the economic challenges, the competition to develop new biologics is intense. Numerous nimble new biotechnology companies—by whatever definition of the admittedly vague category—are competing with the drug industry to develop biologic agents. These new companies often have deep expertise focused on specific areas of biologic research. As a result, these companies produce far more biotech products than the major pharmaceutical companies do. For example, a 2006 PhRMA survey listed 418 biotechnology medicines as under development. The survey indicated only 56 of the biotechnology medicines had a major pharmaceutical company as sole sponsor.[46] The survey listed another 21 medicines as jointly sponsored by a big pharma company and a biotech. The report suggests that, at most, the 12 largest pharmaceutical companies were participating in the development of about 18% of new biologic compounds. Major pharma companies played a somewhat larger role with respect to approved biotech products. The report listed major companies as sole sponsor on 37%. Wharton professors Sean Nicholson and Patricia Danzon found alliances between pharma companies and biotechs were responsible for 38% of the 691 approvals from 1963 to 1999.[47] Heavy reliance on collaborative development of biologics suggests that the major pharma companies will often have to divide any revenues generated.

The new biologics are thus more expensive to develop, may reach smaller markets because of genetic targeting, and may often force companies to divide revenues with development partners. Although the genetics revolution offers boundless scientific possibilities, the economics of biologics will intensify pressures to reduce development costs.

Globalization, Costs, and Competition

The global drug industry is already trying to reduce development costs through outsourcing, a cost-reduction strategy that has swept modern industries. The drug industry has shifted many development activities to geographies with lower costs, especially to emerging economies such as those in India, China, and Eastern Europe. Since technological advances have simplified global communications, much of the planet now has the potential to host laboratory facilities and serve as a recruiting ground for patients to participate in clinical studies (time zone differences and the difficulty of face-to-face contact remain issues). The primary drivers of expanding the research universe to new geographies are cost and patient availability. Diverse genetic backgrounds, cultures, standards of care, and other local differences have not stemmed the tide of outsourcing.

While pharma giants downsize elsewhere, their operations in China are booming:

> The combination of desperation outside China and promise within has convinced almost every big pharmaceutical player, including Roche, Novartis, GlaxoSmithKline, Eli Lilly and Pfizer, to collectively invest hundreds of millions of US dollars into research operations there over the past two to three years. The companies are somewhat cagey about how much they are investing at a time when they are laying off employees elsewhere, and when there is no guarantee of a return. But Kenneth Chien, an expert in cardiovascular medicine and an adviser to several large drug and biotechnology firms working in China, calls it "Basel on steroids," referring to the throng of pharmaceutical companies in Switzerland.[48]

A recent PricewatershouseCoopers report finds that Big Pharma companies rank China and India as the best locations for outsourcing in Asia, followed by Korea and Taiwan. Among reasons for increased pharma outsourcing to Asia, the report cites the growing numbers of highly educated scientific professionals, declining concerns about intellectual property issues, and the availability of large patient populations for clinical testing.[49]

There is no denying the business case for doing the same work, whether drug discovery or clinical testing, in a much less expensive setting. The geographic regions involved do indeed offer much lower costs. Starting salaries for life-sciences Ph.Ds. trained in the United States are $8,000 to $10,000 per year in China, far less than U.S. labs pay such Ph.Ds.[50] Employing a chemist in India costs $60,000 vs. $250,000–$300,000 in the United

States. What is more, India is producing 120,000 chemists and chemical engineers each year.[51]

The trend to conducting clinical studies in new geographic regions is probably most obvious with the testing of oncology products. Until a decade ago, such testing largely took place in the United States. However, patient availability is the most common chokepoint on the speed of clinical research projects. Since cultural issues generally do not affect oncology projects (unlike Alzheimer's trials involving cognitive assessments), oncology trials are good candidates for relocation to areas with lower costs. Many low-cost areas are fertile recruiting grounds because large populations of oncology patients may ordinarily have limited access to chemotherapy. The combination of lower costs and high patient availability drove the shift to Eastern European sites for clinical studies of new oncology treatments over the past decade. Today, it is unusual to perform large-scale oncology programs entirely in the United States. An even larger shift of oncology studies to low-cost areas seems inevitable.

When Offshoring Comes Home

Although globalization presents some attractive possibilities for major pharma companies, it also introduces new challenges. In the long term, globalization seems likely to speed the emergence of new competitors from developing countries. Ultimately, these new competitors will operate their own robust drug development programs with enormous cost advantages. For cost reasons, drug companies already manufacture many drugs in less developed countries, including drugs primarily sold in the developed world. Indian drug firms are taking steps to ensure that their operations comply with FDA regulations, partly as a basis for sales of generic drugs in the United States. However, FDA compliance will also make it easier for Indian companies to bring their own novel compounds to the U.S. market. The labor forces in India and China are receiving on-the-job training in drug development because Western pharmaceutical companies are using growing numbers of Indian and Chinese personnel in their development projects, taking advantage of the pool of highly educated workers with lower salary demands than their Western counterparts. In addition, selective back-recruitment of native researchers who have worked for years as core members of Western pharma companies is proving a ready source of scientific and managerial leadership to propel this competitive evolution.

It would be foolhardy to believe that new low-cost competitors in emerging economies will pass up the enormous business opportunity presented by a global market with high demand, high prices, and high profits. The global drug market seems ripe for price competition driven by countries with significant and growing intellectual capital and a much lower cost structure. Both China and India have large and expanding domestic markets for drugs, an important source of revenue to drive expansion into development of novel compounds. Both countries are major drug exporters as well. China was already exporting $3.5 billion in Western medicines in 2004.[52]

China's interest in developing novel drugs is growing, and China is investing accordingly. The CEO of a company that sells technologies for biotech research says China has "one of the most developed sets of scientific communities that we see outside the United States and is really quite strong in terms of agricultural biotech and gene therapy."[53]

India's Ministry of Science and Technology has stated the goal of becoming a global leader. To that end, the Ministry noted the need for "a shift in the approach of pharmaceutical industry away from manufacturing only known drugs through innovative process routes to discovering and commercializing new molecules."[54] Established firms like Dr. Reddy's, Ranbaxy, and Sun Pharma have growing programs to develop new therapeutic compounds. According to an Ernst & Young report, there are at least 60 new compounds in development by 12 Indian pharmaceutical companies.[55] To be sure, India faces obstacles in advancing to the forefront of drug research, including consistently meeting global standards for good clinical practice (GCP) in clinical trials.[56] At this stage, Indian firms often make partnership deals to have their novel compounds marketed in specific regions by major global pharmaceutical companies. However, the long-term strategy is to make Indian companies robust competitors in the global pharmaceutical industry, leveraging the lower cost and ample supply of scientific expertise in India. This is particularly sobering in the United States, given the steady decline in U.S. nationals pursuing basic science careers at both the graduate and undergraduate levels.

As for clinical development capabilities, both India and China are experiencing rapid growth in the number of active investigators in drug development (Table 1-2). The cost of conducting a phase I clinical trial in China has been reported as anywhere from only 15% of U.S. costs for a phase I trial and 20% of U.S. costs for a phase II trial[57] to less than 50% for phase I and less than 60% of U.S. costs for phases II and III.[58] Total drug development costs in India are 30%–50% lower than in the United States.[59]

Dispersing research operations to low-cost regions undeniably provides substantial savings. However, working across continents, time zones, and cultures inevitably increases the difficulty of managing trials. The problem of managing at a distance is more acute when a study sponsor has reservations about the experience and ability of staff in a new geographic region to provide the quality of GCP essential for clinical studies that provide the basis for successful regulatory submissions. Far-flung, cross-cultural operations may reduce some costs, but they also increase the challenge of managing development programs.

Table 1-2. The number of active clinical investigators developing new drugs in China and India is growing at annual rates of 24% and 18%, respectively.

Country	Number of Active Investigators (2004)	Annual Growth Rate (1999–2004)
North America	28,208	8%
Latin America	240	11%
China	160	24%
India	124	18%
Japan	1,486	6%
Western Europe	8,683	7%
Central and East Europe	327	15%

Source: Tufts Center for the Study of Drug Development 2006, from IMS Health and FDA 2005 data.

More importantly, moving work abroad does nothing to address the fundamental inefficiency of the current approach to clinical research. Inefficiency is inefficiency regardless of the nationality and location of the people involved. For the present, moving clinical operations to regions of lower cost partially relieves the heavy burden of inefficient processes. However, after industry players have completed the offshoring rush, the competition will again come down to how efficiently each player can perform essential tasks. This is especially true as market forces, including greater demands by Western sponsors, predictably shrink differential labor rates and narrow the cost gap. Thus, although outsourcing is an intelligent response to the industry's high development costs and poor productivity, it is at best a short-term solution. At worst, outsourcing places a Band-Aid on a large and growing sore that threatens its host.

The High Risk of Current Development Practices

Improving the efficiency of clinical research is essential if the drug industry is to thrive in an era that seems likely to have fewer blockbusters, the challenging economics of individualized medicine, and formidable new low-cost competitors from emerging countries. Furthermore, lowering development costs would enable the industry to reduce drug prices (or at the very least moderate increases) and defuse public hostility without destroying the profits that fuel research and reward investors.

The risks of continuing current development practices are enormous. Negative attitudes toward the drug industry suggest that the public may be receptive to a variety of proposals to control the cost of prescription drugs.

A familiar proposal modeled on practices in the United Kingdom would establish a single-payer health insurance system and a regulatory body to evaluate medicines not just for efficacy, but for cost-effectiveness as well, thus excluding medicines deemed too expensive from insurance coverage. Another proposal calls for radical restructuring of the entire drug industry, establishing two separate industries. One industry would perform R&D; the other would market drugs. Stan Finkelstein and Peter Temin of the Massachusetts Institute of Technology argue that such a step is necessary:

> The crisis is real. Drug prices are high and getting higher. For those fortunate enough to have health insurance, co-payments are rising, too. Money—whether it has to do with spending it or making it—is an obstacle to getting needed medicines.[60]

Finkelstein and Temin see dividing the industry as the solution: "By separating the risks of drug discovery and development from the chances inherent in marketing medicines, we can cut the Gordian knot that ties together high drug prices and the promise of new drugs." A public nonprofit drug development corporation would acquire new drugs from the companies that develop them and transfer the rights to market the drugs to other companies.

Economic Consequences of Faster Clinical Development

Improved efficiency in clinical development reduces development costs, speeds market entry, and increases revenues and profits. More efficient research and management processes could not only reduce development timelines and the direct costs of conducting studies, but also identify less promising candidates earlier, reducing expenditures on futile projects. Reducing development timelines goes hand in hand with reducing costs (Figure 1-10). For example, a 10% reduction in development time saves 7% of capitalized costs. Cutting development time in half would produce savings of approximately $350 million in total capitalized costs for a typical clinical development project.[61]

Thriving in a New Era

The industry's problems clearly reflect an inability to produce novel products in reasonable time and at reasonable cost. The major reason for this reality is inefficiency in clinical testing, the most costly, time consuming, and risky portion of drug development. The inadequacy of the current approach and the lack of innovation point inevitably to the need for change in strategic thinking. The status quo, it is clear, will condemn the industry to continuation of its recent slump.

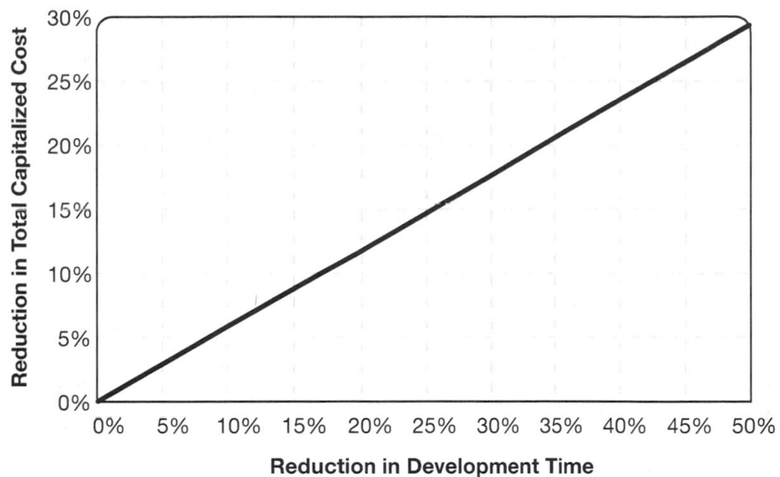

Figure 1-10. Reducing development time by one-half would reduce average per-drug R&D costs by almost 30%, saving an average of more than $350 million. Source: DiMasi 2002.[61]

Although the drug industry's challenges seem daunting, a closer look provides cause for optimism. The root of the industry's problems is clearly the inability to produce novel products in reasonable time and at reasonable cost. It is equally clear that clinical trials consume most of the time and expense of drug development. However, few recognize that already available tools and techniques can enable the industry to streamline clinical trials and reach decision points faster and more efficiently.

The balance of this book discusses the concepts, principles, and specific techniques that will enable the drug industry to improve efficiency and reduce costs. Collectively, these items define adaptive research, an approach that allows midcourse changes based on data collected during trials.

The convergence of communications and computing trends makes the use of adaptive methods in clinical trials not just possible, but practical. Furthermore, the economic pressures on sponsors to improve the development process mandate the application of such technologies. Fundamentally, the adaptive approach involves bringing the tools and techniques of clinical research in line with those long exploited by other modern, efficient industries. There is little doubt that the companies that effectively implement such tools and techniques in drug development will enjoy distinct advantages over companies that do not. Similarly, investors stand to profit from backing companies that can save millions by taking a shorter path to the marketplace or identifying nonviable drugs sooner.

Shorter timelines can greatly reduce development costs. Typical timelines are long indeed. A retrospective study of 168 drugs approved in the period 1994–2002 found a median total post-IND (investigational new drug) development time of 6.3 years. The study found clinical trials consumed 5.1 years, or 81% of the post-IND development time.[62] However, Joseph DiMasi, director of economic analysis for the Tufts Center for the Study of Drug Development, has stated that since 2002 development times have increased.[63] A January 2009 report indicated that average combined times for clinical development and approval are around eight years despite the FDA's success in reducing average approval time to 1.1 years.[64] Based on this information, seven years seems a reasonable estimate for the length of a typical clinical development program. Assume that this includes everything from the first testing in humans through completion of confirmatory studies and preparation of regulatory submissions (Figure 1-11).

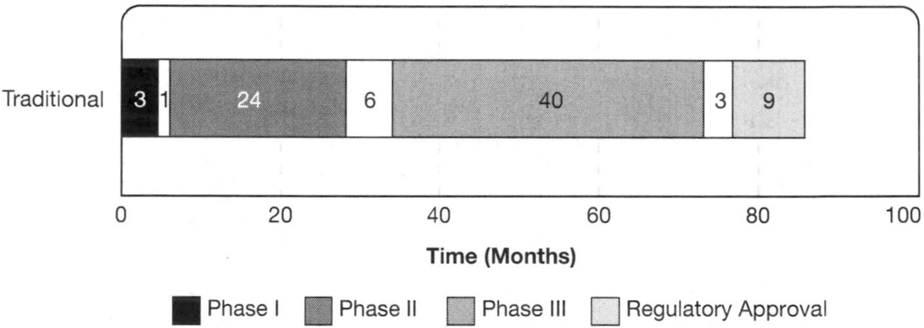

Figure 1-11. A clinical development program typically takes more than seven years from inception to the completion of regulatory submissions. The numbers below each segment indicate duration in months. White indicates between-phase pauses.

Source: Health Decisions, Inc. Used by permission.

For those laboring in the field, such timelines have seemed to lengthen in recent years, leaving the impression that there is little chance of accelerating clinical development. This impression is mistaken. This book will demonstrate principles and techniques that can reduce typical timelines by 25% or more.

Companies that lead the way to more efficient clinical development will reap huge rewards. Laggards will find that adhering to inefficient development practices progressively weakens their competitive standing. Once their descent begins, it will likely prove difficult to recover. On the other hand, industry-wide adoption of a more efficient approach to clinical research could provide enormous benefits. Most dramatically, it could allow the industry to break the dangerous cycle of introducing important new medicines at prices that infuriate the public and shatter the budgets of insurers, businesses that provide health insurance for employees, and individual patients. If that cycle continues, the public may demand radical changes in the status, structure, and role of the drug industry—changes in which the industry would have no voice. Breaking the cycle through greater efficiency could allow the industry to remain in control of its own destiny while also better serving the world's health needs. The principles, technologies, and techniques for breaking the cycle are available. There is no time to lose.

References

1 Go A, Lee W, Yang J, Lo J, Gurwitz J. Statin therapy and risks for death and hospitalization in chronic heart failure. JAMA 2006;296:2105–11.

2 Department of Health and Human Services (US), Food and Drug Administration. Consumer update: celebrating the successes of the Orphan Drug Act. Washington (DC): 2008 Feb 8 [cited Aug 3, 2008]; [about two screens]. Available from: http://www.fda.gov/consumer/updates/oda020808.html.

3 Diabetes. World Health Organization. Geneva: Sept 2006 (Fact Sheet No. 312). Available from: http://www.who.int/mediacentre/factsheets/fs312/en/.

4 Susman E. Analysis: HIV life expectancy now normal. United Press International. Toronto: Aug 25, 2006. Available from: http://www.terradaily.com/reports/HIV_Life_Expectancy_Now_Normal_999.html.

5 Bates S, Weitz J. New anticoagulants: beyond heparin, low-molecular-weight heparin and warfarin. Br J Pharmacol 2005;144:1017–28.

6 Pfizer Inc. annual reports 2001-2007 New York; available from: http://www.pfizer.com/investors/financial_reports/financial_reports.jsp.

7 Morrow D. Warner-Lambert recovers from $7 billion scare. New York Times. Apr 15, 1998. Available from: http://query.nytimes.com/gst/fullpage.html?res=940CE0DF163CF936A25757C0A96E958260&sec=&spon=&pagewanted=2.

8 Pharmaceutical industry profile 2008. Washington (DC): Pharmaceutical Research and Manufacturers of America; Mar 2008. p. ii.

9 Pharma 2020: the vision; which path will you take? New York: PricewaterhouseCoopers LLP. 2007, p. 6. Available from: http://www.pwc.com/extweb/pwcpublications.nsf/docid/91BF330647FFA402852572F2005ECC22.

10 Pharmaceutical Industry Profile 2008. Washington (DC): Pharmaceutical Research and Manufacturers of America; Mar 2008; Pharmaceutical Industry Profile 2006. Washington (DC): Mar 2006; Food and Drug Administration Center for Drug Evaluation and Research. Available from: http://www.fda.gov/AboutFDA/WhatWeDo/History/ProductRegulation/SummaryofNDAAprovalsReceipts1938tothepresent/ucm2006085.htm, accessed October 31, 2009.

11 Rx R&D myths: the case against the drug industry's R&D scare card. Washington (DC): Public Citizen; Jul 23, 2001. Available from: http://www.citizen.org/documents/rd-myths.pdf

12 The economics of TB drug development. New York: Global Alliance for TB Drug Development; Oct 2001. Available from: http://www.tballiance.org/newscenter/publications.php.

13 DiMasi J, Hansen R, Grabowski H. Assessing claims about the cost of new drug development: a critique of the Public Citizen and TB Alliance reports. Tufts Center for the Study of Drug Development. Boston: Nov 1, 2004. Available from: http://csdd.tufts.edu/_documents/www/Doc_231_45_735.pdf.

14 DiMasi J, Hansen R, Grabowski H. The price of innovation: new estimates of drug development costs. J Health Econ. 2003;22:151–85.

15 CNNMoney [Internet] Slud M. Pfizer shareholders OK deal. Apr 27, 2000 [cited Aug 3, 2008]. Available from: http://money.cnn.com/2000/04/27/companies/pfizer/.

16 Berenson A. End of drug trial is a big loss for Pfizer. New York Times. Dec 4, 2006. Available from: http://www.nytimes.com/2006/12/04/health/04pfizer.html.

17 Krauskopf L, Hirschler B. Pfizer shares plunge after cholesterol drug fails. Reuters News Service, New York/London: Dec 4, 2006.

18 Saul S. Release of generic Lipitor is delayed. New York Times. June 19, 2008.

19 Sorkin AR, Wilson D. Pfizer agrees to pay $68 billion for rival drug maker Wyeth. New York Times. Jan 25, 2009.

20 Tansey B. When clinical trial results just say 'no.' San Francisco Chronicle. Mar 11, 2007. Available from: http://www.sfgate.info/cgi-bin/article.cgi?f=/c/a/2007/03/11/BUGC2OHQJ21.DTL&type=chart.

21 Pear R. Spending rise for health care and prescription drugs slows. New York Times. Jan 5, 2009.

22 Fingertip Formulary Insights [Internet]. Glen Rock, NJ: Sept 2007 [cited Aug 3, 2008]; pp. 1–5. Available from: http://www.fingertipformulary.com/newsletter/2007-09/pdf/Insights_Sept07.pdf.

23 Norman P. Generic competition 2007 to 2011 — the impact of patent expiries on sales of major drugs. Summary. Urch Publishing, London: Feb 2007 [cited Aug 3, 2008]. Available from: http://www.urchpublishing.com/publications/general/generic_competition_2011_00.html.

24 Goodman M. Market Watch: Pharma industry performance metrics: 2007–2012E. Nat Rev Drug Discov. 2008;7:795.

25 Simons J. Pfizer's puzzle. The Fortune 500; Pfizer No. 31. Fortune. Apr 17, 2006. pp. 152–53.

26 Garnier J-P. Rebuilding the R&D engine in big pharma. Harvard Business Review. 2008;86:68–76.

27 IMS Health [Internet]. Global pharmaceutical sales, 2000–2007. Mar 28, 2008 [cited Aug 3, 2008]; Norwalk (CT). Available from: http://www.imshealth.com/portal/site/imshealth/menuitem.a46c6d4df3db4b3d88f611019418c22a/?vgnextoid=67a89df4609e9110VgnVCM10000071812ca2RCRD&cpsextcurrchannel=1.

28 Loftus, P. US drug market faces down year. Wall Street Journal. Apr 23, 2009.

29 Adams C, Brantner V. Estimating the cost of new drug development: is it really $802 million? Health Aff. 2006;25:420–28.

30 Tollman P, Guy P, Altshuler J, Flanagan A, Steiner M. A revolution in R&D: how genomics and genetics are transforming the biopharmaceutical industry. Boston (MA): Boston

Consulting Group. Nov 2001. 60 p. Available from: http://www.bcg.com/publications/files/eng_genomicsgenetics_rep_11_01.pdf [cited Aug 3, 2008].

31 Gilbert J, Henske P, Singh A. Rebuilding big pharma's business model. Windhover Information Inc. In Vivo, the Business and Medicine Report 2003;21:73–80.

32 DiMasi J, Grabowski H. The cost of pharmaceutical R&D: is biotech different? Managerial Decis Econ. 2007;28:469–79.

33 Tufts Center for the Study of Drug Development. Boston (MA): Citing Boston Consulting Group, 1993; Peck, Food and Drug Law J, 1997; Parexel, 2002.

34 Growing protocol design complexity stresses investigators, volunteers. Tufts CSDD Impact Report. Tufts Center for the Study of Drug Development. Boston (MA): 2008;10. Summary available from: http://csdd.tufts.edu/_documents/www/Doc_309_65_893.pdf.

35 Getz K. Protocol design trends and their effect on clinical trial performance. Regul Affairs J - Pharma. 2008;19:315–6.

36 Prescription drug trends. Kaiser Family Foundation. Menlo Park (CA). May 2007. (Fact Sheet No.: 3057-06.) Available from: http://www.kff.org/rxdrugs/upload/3057_06.pdf.

37 Prescription drug trends. Kaiser Family Foundation. Menlo Park (CA). Oct 2004. (Fact Sheet No.: 3057-03.) Available from: http://www.kff.org/rxdrugs/upload/Prescription-Drug-Trends-October-2004-UPDATE.pdf.

38 Bazell R. Strange medicine: why are the new cancer drugs so expensive? [Internet] Slate. Jun 23, 2004. Available from: http://www.slate.com/id/2102844/.

39 Mayer R. Two steps forward in the treatment of colorectal cancer. NEJM 2004;350:2406–2508.

40 Kolata G, Pollack A. The evidence gap: costly cancer drug offers hope, but also a dilemma. New York Times. July 6, 2008. Available from: http://www.nytimes.com/2008/07/06/health/06avastin.html?_r=1&oref=slogin.

41 Martinez B, Johnson A. Drug makers, hospitals raise prices. Wall Street Journal. Apr 15, 2009.

42 Department of Labor (US), Bureau of Labor Statistics. Consumer price index summary. Washington (DC). Apr 15, 2009. Available from: http://www.bls.gov/news.release/cpi.nr0.htm.

43 Views on prescription drugs and the pharmaceutical industry. Kaiser Health Poll Report. Kaiser Family Foundation, Menlo Park (CA). Jan/Feb 2005. Available from: http://www.kff.org/healthpollreport/feb_2005/index.cfm.

44 Views on prescription drugs and the pharmaceutical industry. Kaiser Public Opinion Spotlight. Kaiser Family Foundation. Menlo Park (CA). Updated Apr 2008. Available from: http://www.kff.org/spotlight/rxdrugs/upload/Rx_Drugs.pdf.

45 Trusheim M, Berndt E, Douglas F. Impact of genetic diagnostics on drug development strategy. Nat Rev Drug Discov. 2007;6:287–93.

46 2006 Report: Medicines in development, biotechnology. Pharmaceutical Research and Manufacturers of America. Washington (DC): July 2006. Available from: http://www.phrma.org/files/Biotech%202006.pdf.

47 Danzon P, McCulloch J, Nicholson S. Biotech-pharma alliances as a signal of asset and firm quality. J Bus. 2002;78:1433–64.

48 Cyranoski D. Pharmaceutical future: Made in China? Nature. 2008;455:1168.

49 The changing dynamics of pharma outsourcing in Asia: Are you readjusting your sights? PricewatershouseCoopers. 2008.

50 Dolan K. The drug research war. Forbes.com. May 4, 2008. Available from: http://www.forbes.com/2004/05/28/cz_kd_0528outsourcing.html.

51 White paper on Indian pharma industry quest for global leadership. Cygnus Business Consulting & Research. Hyderabad, India: Nov 14, 2006. [cited Aug 3, 2008] Available from: http://www.cygnusindia.com/white_papers.asp.

52 Fishman T. China Inc. New York: Scribner; 2005. p. 223.

53 Fishman 2005. p. 118. Quoted from: Lucier G. China as an emerging regional and technology power: implications for US economic and security interests. Testimony before the US-China Economic and Security Review Commission. Washington (DC): Feb 12–13, 2004. [Cited Aug 3, 2008] Available from: http://www.uscc.gov/hearings/2004hearings/written_testimonies/04_02_12wrts/lucier.htm.

54 Drugs & pharmaceutical research. Scientific programmes. Technology development. Department of Science & Technology (India). New Delhi. [cited Aug 3, 2008] Available from: http://dst.gov.in/scientific-programme/td-drugs.htm.

55 Palnitkar U. The Indian pharmaceutical industry: promises and perils. Pharma Focus Asia. 2007;3(4). Pharmafocusasia.com [Internet].Ochre Media Pvt. Ltd. Hyderabad, India. Available from: http://www.pharmafocusasia.com/strategy/indian_pharma_promises.htm.

56 Jayaraman KS. Firms discovering reality of clinical research in India. Nat Rev Drug Discov. 2006;5:6.

57 Reymond E. China lives up to outsourcing hype. Outsourcing-pharma.com. Jan 16, 2007. [cited Aug 3, 2008]; [about 2 screens]. Available from: http://www.outsourcing-pharma.com/Clinical-Development/China-lives-up-to-outsourcing-hype.

58 Behera D, Shindikar A. Clinical trials: Growing opportunities for India. Pharmainfo.net. [Cited Aug 3, 2008] Available from: http://www.pharmainfo.net/reviews/clinical-trials-growing-opportunities-india.

59 Rahul Das D, Sharma A. Destination: India. Drug Discovery & Development. Aug 1, 2007. [cited Aug 3, 2008] Available from: http://www.dddmag.com/destination-india.aspx

60 Finkelstein S, Temin P. Reasonable Rx: Solving the drug price crisis. Upper Saddle River, NJ: FT Press; 2008.

61 DiMasi J. The value of improving the productivity of the drug development process: faster times and better decisions. Pharmacoeconomics. 2002;20 Suppl 3:1–10.

62 Keyhani S, Diener-West M, Powe N; AcademyHealth. Meeting (2005: Boston). Abstr AcademyHealth Meet. 2005; 22: abstract no. 3676. Available from: http://gateway.nlm.nih.gov/MeetingAbstracts/ma?f=103623139.html.

63 Prescription drug development time has decreased over 10 years, study finds. Medical News Today. Mar 10, 2006. Available from: http://www.medicalnewstoday.com/articles/39161.php.

64 Outlook 2009. Tufts Center for the Study of Drug Development. Boston: Jan 2009. Available from: http://csdd.tufts.edu/InfoServices/OutlookReports.asp.

— Chapter 2 —

Defining and Extending the Adaptive Approach

The Adaptive Concept

The word "adaptive" broadly means having the flexibility to change while something is in progress. Our daily lives exemplify the adaptive approach: when circumstances change, we consider changing our behavior. We assess circumstances based on a variety of inputs, often including information technology, to help decide on appropriate responses. For example, if an accident blocks our usual route to work, we find an alternate, perhaps using real-time traffic information from a dashboard global positioning system (GPS). This is how we do just about everything in life—by incorporating new information with existing experience and knowledge, we make adjustments to maximize our chances of success.

Efficient modern businesses operate in the same way. They achieve greatest efficiency and productivity through "tight" management—relying on a continuous stream of up-to-the-minute information for quick recognition and correction of deviations from an efficient course. For a variety of reasons, including sheer complexity and geographic dispersion, modern businesses rely on computational and communications systems for a continuously updated flow of electronic data. The same electronic tools also provide continuous analysis that transforms raw data into meaningful information. A manager's experience and judgment translate information into knowledge, allowing timely decisions to optimize operations. This process continues in a cycle, repeatedly measuring the effects of changes against desired outcomes. The continuous cycle of measurement, assessment, and intervention enables precise management.

Knowledge, Time, and Decision Making

In contrast to the model of continuous measurement and refinement, conventional clinical studies present a "black box" that intentionally impedes the flow of information. Companies try to conduct efficient studies, acquiring the desired information with minimal timelines and costs. However, conventional practice presents major obstacles. There are strict limits on access to data collected during a study. On a strategic level, study and program managers usually know very little until study completion. Prior experience and best estimates, often guesses, guide decisions. Managers can only hope actual study data will closely match planning estimates for parameters that determine the ability to detect a difference between test drug and comparator. Large studies may allow independent safety oversight groups to examine data collected during a trial, but many trials lack even this restricted view of data. As with study data, managers have access to few if any performance metrics to track key activities such as enrollment and ensuring data accuracy. In summary, limited access to data and the absence of measures tracking progress during studies severely handicap managers.

Like Christopher Columbus sailing to discover a new route to Asia, study managers begin with limited information and set off in the general direction of what they hope to find. Like Columbus, study managers receive very little information along the way. Columbus missed the riches of Asia by thousands of miles, making landfall on a Bahamian island that offered no rewards to cover the costs of the voyage. Modern clinical research often misses the mark for the same reason that prevented Columbus from reaching his desired destination—want of information to track progress and allow course corrections. This is the single greatest cause of inefficiency in clinical research and explains why so many studies represent wasted investments.

For both design and operational aspects of clinical studies, the lack of access to information tracking study progress amounts to a "well of ignorance." (See Figure 2-1.) In some cases, information becomes available too late to be of value. In other cases, information is lacking altogether. Indeed, Figure 2-1 may overstate the amount of information that comes too late and understate the amount that never comes at all. For example, although enrollment rates greatly influence a study's duration and cost, formal processes to assess and refine enrollment strategies are virtually nonexistent. Rather than identifying and correcting problems, the current approach often ensures the continuation of inefficient or futile practices until study's end. The back-of-the-envelope management that may suffice in a small trial has no chance against the complexities of a typical contemporary study involving multiple sites and a large patient population.

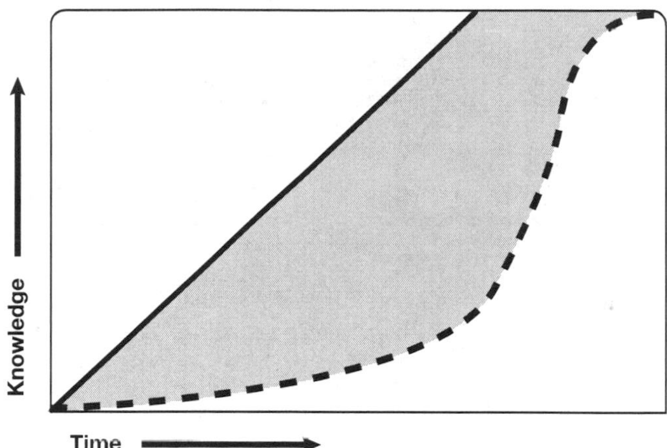

Figure 2-1. In a conventional clinical trial, there is a lag between the generation of information (solid line) and its availability to study managers (dashed line), casting managers into a well of ignorance. Such delays preclude timely corrective actions.

Source: Health Decisions, Copyright 2004. Used by permission.

Delayed acquisition of study knowledge impairs management of entire programs as well as individual studies. Since all knowledge from a study usually becomes available to program managers only at the very end, the acquisition of knowledge within the program proceeds in large steps separated by long intervals (Figure 2-2). This stepwise process is a slow, expensive and unnecessarily risky way to acquire knowledge. Every researcher responsible for assessing one study before progressing to the next has experienced the anxiety that builds as the study nears its conclusion. The clinical team rushes to resolve remaining queries, managers lock the database, and statisticians work intensively at their computers. Then mountains of printouts start landing on the designated researcher's desk. Each new mountain raises issues that require further analysis. Any steps to implement the next study must await the researcher's analysis and interpretation. The ticking clock undermines the thoughtful, systematic team approach appropriate for any complex, high-stakes decision, increasing the risk of error. Suboptimal decisions may jeopardize subsequent studies, delay development, and endanger investments.

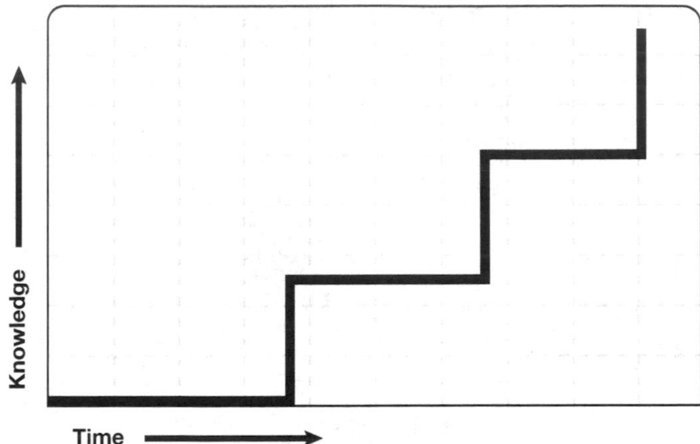

Figure 2-2. Conventional development programs acquire knowledge at long intervals defined by individual studies, with no knowledge of key outcomes until the end of each study. Then great quantities of data suddenly become available for analysis and interpretation.

Source: Health Decisions, Copyright 2006. Used by permission.

The Value of Early Knowledge

Clinical research has long allowed consideration of protocol amendments based on unanticipated trial developments. Increasing reliance on interim analysis reflects an understanding of the importance of acquiring knowledge earlier and using it to improve the efficiency of clinical studies. However, protocol amendments are narrow, ad hoc responses to the unforeseen. Interim analysis not only has a narrow focus, but also allows numerous unknown changes to accumulate until the time for the analysis comes.

The notion of acquiring earlier knowledge as a basis for improving efficiency has the potential for wide application. The most common application provides for early termination for futility. The same approach can also sometimes allow completing studies more efficiently by correcting problems in both study design and operations. One technique for correcting a design issue addresses sample size, the single greatest determinant of study costs. Study planners calculate the number of test subjects required based on estimates of parameters such as the magnitude of treatment effect and variability of data. Only the data actually collected during the study can determine the correct values for these parameters. If the actual value for the treatment effect differs significantly from the estimate, the sample size will be incorrect, perhaps compromising the study's ability to demonstrate a difference between the test drug and the comparator. Sample-size reestimation uses data collected during the study to increase sample size and preserve statistical significance or decrease sample size and reduce study costs.

Adjusting a Study Design

One enormous study adjusted at midcourse for higher variability of the treatment effect than anticipated, preventing a massive effort involving tens of thousands of subjects from going to waste. The study was testing the efficacy of a new herpes zoster vaccine. Planners estimated that the study would require 440 evaluable cases of herpes zoster in order to detect a 60% reduction in pain score with 97% power. However, the variability measured after the first 200 evaluable cases showed that the study would actually need 750 evaluable cases to detect the difference as required. The study increased sample size to approximately 37,200 patients. As a result the study produced results that allowed the vaccine, Merck's Zostavax, to win approval.[1,2] Chapter 3 provides additional information on how the Zostavax study adjusted sample size.

Adjusting Enrollment Strategy

The story with many enrollment issues is the same as with adjusting sample size based on data collected during a study—knowing sooner makes all the difference between missing enrollment targets and meeting timelines. Continuous tracking of data on reasons for screen failures or success rates for different recruitment techniques can allow adjustments in enrollment strategy that keep the study on schedule. For example, enrollment for one sexually transmitted disease (STD) study was lagging far behind schedule. Study managers used recruitment data for individual sites to identify one site that was successfully recruiting enough patients. The successful site was using a recruitment strategy that the study team and the other sites had never considered. That site manager thought individuals at risk for STD might frequent nightclubs. The site was getting excellent results from posting notices in nightclub restrooms. When study managers helped other sites adopt the same strategy, the study completed enrollment in 9 months, 2 months ahead of schedule. Recruitment at the initial slow rate would have required 18 months to enroll enough patients. The study's rapid adaptation of enrollment strategy based on data collected during the study cut the enrollment period in half.* Chapter 5 provides more detailed information about adaptive enrollment in this STD study.

These examples show how access to vital information during a study can boost efficiency. Both examples require the same basic process—timely data collection during a trial, access to trial data while the trial is in progress, analysis that identifies a problem, and action to correct the problem. Al-

*Health Decisions, Inc. conducted the study.

though for many in the industry the term "adaptive research" refers only to midcourse changes in study designs, the STD study described above shows how applying the same adaptive principles to study operations provides similar benefits. For this reason, it makes sense to extend the definition of adaptive research to include midcourse operational changes. Design adaptations have shown the way, but operational adaptations deserve similar recognition as methods of improving the efficiency of clinical research. Neglecting operational adaptations, however mundane they may seem alongside sophisticated techniques for design adaptations, will prevent the industry from increasing the efficiency of clinical research enough to meet its major challenges. The industry must use the adaptive approach to improve the efficiency of every aspect of clinical studies.

The Spectrum of Design and Operational Adaptations

The adaptive approach can apply equally well to a wide range of design and operational issues based on access to data while studies are in progress. In brief, design adaptations include: sample size reestimation, adaptive randomization (changing the proportion of patients allocated to different study arms to meet such objectives as minimizing patient exposure to ineffective or less safe treatments or balancing covariates across study arms), seamless transition between study phases, adaptive dose ranging to better select doses for subsequent testing, refocusing on responsive subpopulations, and adjusting hypotheses, such as switching from a hypothesis of superiority to one of noninferiority.

The range of potential operational adaptations extends across aspects that greatly affect the efficiency of all clinical trials, whether or not the trials involve design adaptations, including enrollment, site performance, resource allocation, and data management.

Maximizing the Adaptive Approach: Agile Clinical Development

Besides gaining access to data collected during studies, it is imperative to make more extensive use of information technology. Study managers need tools that aid in understanding and using enormous quantities of data quickly enough to take advantage of what has been learned at any point, whether to optimize study designs or operations. The ability to assess new data and respond at frequent intervals is essential for effective management of complex trials, often multinational, with many components that must mesh to produce timely, reliable data. The shorter the interval between responses, the better. The ideal is not just to shorten intervals, but for study managers to receive information continuously and respond whenever necessary. Management based on continuous measurements of study progress defines the ideal of agile clinical development. Optimal implementation of adaptive methods requires using the agile approach to managing studies.

Five key principles underlie agile clinical development:

- Measure performance in real time.
- Provide the right information to the right person as quickly as possible.
- Make timely decisions, based on that information.
- Organize work in lean processes.
- Match technology with tasks.

Together with the capacity to adapt both study designs and operations, these five principles enable adaptive methods and allow much more responsive and efficient management of clinical studies. The five principles behind agile clinical development have proved their value in the modernization of other major industries, beginning with automobile manufacturing but more recently including service industries as well.[3]

Measure Performance in Real Time

In 1911, Frederick Taylor laid the groundwork for modern management by emphasizing the usefulness of breaking jobs down into fundamental activities and measuring productivity by how many times a worker can perform the same task in a given period of time.[4] Taylor called this approach "scientific management." Ideas for measuring the performance of professionals like those who conduct clinical trials began to appear in 1954 with Peter Drucker's *The Practice of Management*.[5] In 1959, Drucker would coin the term "knowledge workers" for such people.[6] Among his many insights, Drucker introduced the idea of management by objective.

Drucker also asserted the need for managers to establish yardsticks to measure performance of the people they supervised, as expressed in the truism, "If you can't measure it, you can't manage it." Drucker described this basic management need with greater precision: "It should indeed be an invariable practice to supply managers with clear and common measurements in all key areas of a business."[7] Perhaps more importantly, Drucker also emphasized that the measurements must be available in time to allow making any necessary changes; reliable, with attention to margin of error; and clear enough to make discussion and interpretation unnecessary. In short, managers need measurements as a reliable, practical basis for timely decisions.

Like any business, clinical research cannot effectively manage without yardsticks. Most researchers think of accumulating CRF data as the measure of study progress. More precise and useful performance metrics track major activities in the execution of the study itself. These performance metrics are essential for managing studies more efficiently and completing them more quickly. Such performance metrics track activities, including:

- enrollment, which profoundly affects timelines and costs;
- data accuracy, where query rates are a vital measure because each query represents costly rework;
- progress toward database lock, through measures such as number of queries outstanding.

Management of these central issues requires timely, accurate data and rapid analytic tools. Some valuable measures, created in advance, include predefined decision criteria, as in the case of decisions about which dosing arms to discontinue. The need for other measures may not become apparent until the study is in progress, such as measures for tracking a side effect that becomes an issue after study inception. Much discussion about precisely what measures to put in place should take place in the planning stage so that during the study the combination of data and analytics can quickly direct attention where it should go and provide a sound basis for rapid decisions and corrective actions. Relying on performance metrics requires perspective on their limitations and interactions with other considerations in managing studies:

- While information must be both timely and accurate, there are often tradeoffs between these two important attributes.
- Managing some trial activities does not require metrics with a high standard of certainty and precision. The standard of precision depends on the nature, context, and timing of related decisions. To be useful, a metric must be accurate enough to engender confidence in decision-makers, but also provide information in time to make a decision that can have an effect.
- It is sometimes necessary to strike a balance between the certainty and precision of information and the ability to make decisions while they still matter.
- Informational needs may change during a study and metrics may have to change or expand with them.
- Metrics are to improve the effectiveness of management, not to enable countless decisions about minutiae; managers must make judgments about which metrics enable decisions that will truly contribute to greater efficiency.

In some cases, acting on early and imperfect data may be preferable to waiting to ascertain a figure with 100% certainty and an arbitrary number of decimal places; what is important is recognizing the limitations of any data before using it. In a clinical setting, for example, some operational data represents query rates from many different sites. With data of this type, what matters is to understand the general frequency of queries, identify sites that generate markedly more queries, and understand what accounts for higher query rates at particular sites. The goal with such metrics is to recognize problems and trends early on in order to take prompt remedial action. If query rates are high at a couple of sites, that is one piece of information; if query rates exceed expected levels based on previous similar studies, that indicates a different type of problem. The manager's job is to track down what is causing problems and intervene. For example, the reason for a high query rate across all sites might be a poorly worded question on a case report form (CRF), a confusing sequence of items, or a programming error affecting assembly of data from the questionnaire and its transfer into the database.

Both measurement of performance against objectives and more detailed measurements of productivity and quality are essential for effective management of any activity as complex as a clinical trial. While the types of performance metrics useful in managing clinical trials are too numerous to list at this point, a few examples will illustrate the benefits of such metrics.

Metrics in Action

An example of important but commonly overlooked management information regards patient recruitment. This is one of the most important drivers of study cost—over three-quarters of studies fall short of enrollment targets.[8] Delays and other problems in patient recruitment can have a devastating effect on everything from data reliability to efficiency, morale, and stock price. Effective management of clinical trials requires knowing not only how many patients are being successfully recruited, screened, and enrolled at each investigational site but also which specific approaches are working and which are not. Site personnel, generally not trained in management and without incentives to improve, tend to pay little attention to recruitment and enrollment. Sites cannot judge their own performance because they lack a means to compare their approach with that of other sites. Study management devotes surprisingly little attention to recruitment. A good reporting system continuously assesses successes and failures at each stage, allowing managers to identify successful strategies and quickly share these with other sites. This simple strategy can greatly improve recruitment. In the STD study described earlier in "Adjusting Enrollment Strategy," such information and the project manager's initiative allowed enrollment to take off. The only way to know which recruitment techniques are working is to identify all techniques in use and measure results from the outset.

Monitoring rate of screen failures and reasons for screen failures at each site is essential for managing recruitment effectively. For example, when reality proves optimistic inclusion/exclusion criteria too restrictive for practical execution of the study, relaxing some criteria even slightly can sometimes greatly accelerate enrollment. Allowing patients with a half-gram lower hemoglobin level, for example, may be a reasonable trade-off. The issue is establishing criteria before knowing conditions in the field. The ability to track critical enrollment information allows consideration of adjusting criteria. The availability of appropriate metrics can allow management responses such as altering recruitment strategy to find a source of appropriate patients who are less likely to have an attribute associated with screen failure, or even to consider whether one of the inclusion/exclusion criteria presents an insurmountable barrier to recruiting the number of patients needed for the study. Without suitable recruitment metrics, study managers and sponsors can only add more sites and commit more resources, increasing both complexity and costs.

Timely metrics are also indispensable for determining whether to carry out sophisticated adaptations to study design in accordance with predetermined decision rules. There is a strong imperative to make such decisions quickly, but any such decision must rest on accurate data. Combining a design that allows sample-size reestimation and operational arrangements that provide accurate data when needed allows completing the reestimation with only a short interval—optimally, a day or less—between an interim database lock and the availability of the clean data required to perform a reestimation. Effective use of adaptive randomization and dose-finding methods requires even more timely access to information on patient response.

Timely tracking of data queries represents another major opportunity to improve clinical operations. Detailed measures of reasons for queries allow correcting the problems that are causing errors. Since a substantial portion of site activity consists of reworking initial data that contains errors, timely identification of errors and intervention to reduce recurrences reduces site effort, increasing site profit or reducing sponsor expenditures. Furthermore, the measures tracking the capture and validation of patient data by each site allow offering incentives and disincentives based on quality of data and timeliness of data submission and query resolution. Useful measurements include query rate, number of queries outstanding, mean time to query resolution, and number of queries generated for each data field, in all cases both study-wide and by individual investigational site. Such metrics enable study managers to zero in on problems slowing the accumulation of validated information in the study database. Often these metrics allow tracing problems to issues at specific sites or to systemic causes such as CRF design flaws causing high error rates in particular fields. The problems may also reveal the need to improve training of study personnel, whether at a few sites or everywhere. If metrics are available to help identify the nature, scope, and locus of such problems early on, prompt action can greatly accelerate study progress, site closeout, and database lock.

Useful management metrics can relate to anything that affects workflow. This includes elements of recruitment, data capture, the flow of study supplies, the number of on-schedule patient visits at each site, the number of CRFs reviewed by each monitor, parameters that affect statistical power and sample-size calculations, and many other possibilities.

Right Information to the Right Eyes at the Right Time

Some of the inefficiency in today's clinical studies derives from excessive reliance on a top-down management approach, with decision-making power on both major and minor issues focused in the hands of one or a few individuals. The top-down approach dates from an era when data handling and communications moved at a fraction of today's routine speeds. The top-down approach often leads to underutilization of talent, suppression of creativity, and limitations on effective teamwork in many types of organizations.

The top-down approach is anachronistic for several reasons. First, most clinical studies today involve multiple sites, often dispersed around the world. Second, taking advantage of time-sensitive performance metrics tracking many aspects of trial operations requires making far more decisions—too many for a single person. Experience shows that sooner or later the top-down approach transforms key managers into rate-limiting chokepoints. Third, in many cases, the person most directly familiar with operational issues can best understand and act on relevant performance metrics. Finally, the top-down approach inherently magnifies the limitations of those at the top. For all these reasons, top-down management is a handicap in today's environment with rapid computing and communications. The clearest example is in field monitoring, where an in-house team can work far more effectively than a single individual whose particular limitations may reduce efficiency.

The ability to involve a wider group, discussed in *The Wisdom of Crowds*,[9] can allow more reliable, faster decision making. Involving a wider group requires evolution toward a model of distributed management. This does not imply abandoning the notion of central control. Instead, it emphasizes harnessing the entire team to achieve the goals of each study, with the most important decisions still reserved for project leaders and program managers. Managing the complex processes of clinical trials requires the varied expertise and skill of entire study teams. Furthermore, the internet, e-mail, and access controls simplify both wide and targeted sharing of information.

Involving the entire study team in a targeted way not only allows harnessing the strengths of all team members, but also prevents large volumes of performance metrics and study data from overwhelming team members. Having each person pore over an enormous body of data to identify the portion relevant to that person's role wastes time and may lead to inappropriate choices. Instead, study systems and processes should present an appropriate selection of information to each person. For example, the CEO may want to know the projected completion dates of key studies. The head of clinical research may want completion dates for all clinical projects, highlighting those that are behind schedule. The project manager may want to track enrollment, screen failures, and number of patients at each stage of the trial. The CRA will want to know error rates in data submitted, which questions are causing problems, and how many unmonitored fields are at each of her sites. Distributing appropriate information to each member of the study or program team should take into account Drucker's requirement for "self-announcing" measurements. Ideally, important information should appear in a form that makes it easy to identify emerging trends and problems and provides a basis for appropriate action.[7] While systems and processes should attempt to filter information to meet each person's needs, they should also avoid needlessly excluding study staff from more comprehensive information that may prove useful in a variety of ways.

Make Timely Decisions

Metrics are worthless unless managers understand them and make timely decisions to address any problems as they become apparent. The variety of decisions called for depends on what the metrics measure and what insights the data provides. Although this point seems obvious, clinical research has relied for so long on a methodological approach that requires waiting until the end of the trial for access to information that many managers are accustomed to making few if any decisions. Should useful performance metrics suddenly appear, many study managers trained in a hands-off approach would hesitate to consider and act on them. Such trial managers look in on a trial occasionally to see if anything obvious has gone wrong. They are not the vigorous, active managers prized in most modern enterprises and essential for improving the efficiency of clinical trials. Effective study managers must show determination to understand what is going on and to act to ensure the most productive and efficient trial given the realities encountered.

While there are cases that require restricting access to exclude bias, more often there is no good reason to delay access. Careful procedures and restrictions can prevent the wrong eyes from seeing information that might allow bias to creep in. To achieve greater efficiency in clinical research, we need to ensure that we obtain and examine all the information necessary unless there is a specific reason to remain in the dark. Moreover, we should carefully examine whether all study personnel must remain ignorant of all types of information, or whether certain designated individuals, subject to strict controls, can learn specific types of information for management purposes. In the most formal cases of decision making involving early stopping rules or rule-based design adaptations, access to certain information may be confined to a data management committee or an independent statistical service. However, in many cases managers can access the information needed to conduct an efficient trial without jeopardizing integrity or validity.

There is frequently a time imperative on making decisions regarding design adaptations. For example, in rising-dose escalation studies, the cycle time required to make a decision about the next dose cohort needs to be as short as possible, consistent with complete information and deliberation. Decisions on the next dose to administer generally hinge on patient safety data, and systems need to be in place to provide the required information rapidly. In a world where a week or more is the norm for such decisions, current technology enables presentation of this information in hours and shortening the cycle time to one day. With sample-size reestimations, it is important to minimize the interval between interim database lock and the time at which statisticians receive clean data to perform the recalculation. In this instance, prompt data availability can reduce the usual delay of weeks or months to one day.

The technology platform that provides the timely availability of information for decisions regarding design-level adaptations is precisely the same platform that enables operational adaptations. The same platform empowers decision making in both realms. Once the platform is in place, timely decision making becomes possible.

Organize Work in Lean Processes

In the first quarter of 2008, Toyota sold 160,000 more cars than General Motors. GM had been the leading producer since the 1930s. Toyota's ascendancy reflects the triumph of a management approach that focuses on defining processes precisely and optimizing them continuously.[10] Process optimization requires analyzing how to achieve a goal most efficiently, without deference to current practices and preconceptions. Toyota's Taiichi Ohno first described the approach that made Toyota so efficient.[11] Later, James Womack and co-authors named the approach "lean thinking" and explained it to a Western audience.[3,12]

The essence of lean thinking includes clearly identifying the value that operations are intended to create, analyzing the stream of activities that create this value for the end customer, ensuring the continuous flow of the value stream toward the customer, and striving always to improve the efficiency of the value stream and all the activities that feed into it. Lean thinking seeks to banish all effort, time, and expense that are not actually creating value for the customer.

Lean manufacturing supplanted the traditional batch-and-queue approach that long dominated global manufacturing—an approach that still has echoes in the way we conduct clinical studies. Ohno's transformative observation was noticing that performing operations in batches, though more efficient than old craft-like processes, often brought the production process to a halt.[11] Batches waited to be fed to high-speed equipment and afterward waited before entering the next stage of the production process. Ohno focused on organizing work to prevent production from halting, maintaining a continuous forward flow of work and value. Above all, Ohno eliminated any waste or any activity that caused "backflow," the redirection of effort into activities that reversed the value stream. The prime example of backflow is having to rework something done incorrectly the first time. The attitude exemplified in lean thinking is to do things right the first time, maximizing quality and eliminating delays. A further principle of lean thinking is standardizing work procedures, both to reduce the incidence of errors and to allow reliable measures of performance. Measurements of standardized processes can identify problems and provide the information needed for continuous improvement to increase efficiency over time.

The value of the lean approach seems clear in car manufacturing—the car buyer gets an efficient, comfortable, and reliable new vehicle on demand at a good price. At first glance, it is less obvious how lean thinking applies to clinical research. However, lean thinking provides many insights for making clinical research more efficient. The program manager is to a clinical study as the car buyer is to a new car made by Toyota. The value the program manager seeks is accurate, complete, and statistically valid information about the effectiveness and safety of a new drug. The information from early-phase studies must arrive on time and within budget, if not sooner and at lower cost. It must support a decision as to whether to conduct subsequent studies. Information from confirmatory studies must meet the requirements for a regulatory filing and must also meet or beat time and cost requirements. According to lean thinking, the standard for assessing process improvements in clinical research is whether they do in fact contribute to delivering the desired package of accurate, complete and valid information about a new drug on time and within budget or even earlier and at lower cost. The same standard applies to assessing technological tools.

Rework in Clinical Studies

The complexity of clinical studies bears a striking resemblance to the complexity of car manufacturing. A typical car has approximately 10,000 parts, most of them made at external sites and shipped to the factory. The number of permutations and combinations in manufacturing a single car can reach 300,000,000, as in the case of the Volkswagen Golf V.[13] In a typical old factory, it took approximately 25% of total work hours to fix mistakes made earlier. Standard practice allowed flaws to travel all the way to the end of the assembly line, where there was a large rework area.[12] Rework was costly but essential.

Like a car, the report summarizing a clinical study has many parts— thousands or millions of data points collected at many external investigational sites and sent to a central location for processing. The clinical research equivalent of the assembly line is the progression of externally collected data through a process of cleaning, validation, and analysis at the central location. A conventional clinical study devotes 25%–30% of its expenditures to remediation of protocol violations, comparable to the percentage of work old car factories had to devote to fixing problems at the end of the assembly line. However, protocol violations are only one of the kinds of problems that slow clinical trials. Data-entry and transcription errors are also common; this is not surprising considering the number of entries made and continued widespread reliance on hand data entry. Undetected data errors are probably not on a scale that produces erroneous findings, but are enough to muddy the waters, making the difference between a test drug and its comparator more difficult to detect. This increases the number of subjects that trials need and adds to costs and timelines. In some cases, such errors may be systematic and result in erroneous conclusions or even mask safety problems that become apparent later on.

While Toyota corrected problems as soon as they were detected and reduced the percentage of time devoted to rework almost to zero,[12] clinical research has not yet devoted serious attention to preventing as many mistakes as possible as early as possible. Common practice in companies conducting clinical trials today is to take the occurrence of numerous errors for granted, relying on monitors to fix problems after the fact, or simply excluding patients in the event of protocol violations. The query process in clinical studies is an institutionalized way of correcting work that was done wrong the first time—the equivalent of the rework area in an old, inefficient car factory. While the availability of the query process is essential to identify and correct errors and ensure the accuracy of data, making clinical studies more efficient requires minimizing the occurrence of errors by identifying and fixing the root causes as soon as possible. The lean approach's intolerance of repeated errors and focus on continuous process improvement could greatly improve efficiency in clinical research as it has in car manufacturing.

Backflow of Patient Data

The capture of patient data on CRFs and validation of the data for entry into the study database together constitute one of the most essential processes of clinical research. Everybody who works on clinical studies knows how data capture and validation work. While web-based electronic data capture (EDC) offers some improvement over paper and pen, it also introduces needless delays and expenses. Medical professionals at investigational sites are still filling out data on paper patient records. Someone must then transcribe the data onto CRFs by hand. After that, the data remains on paper until somebody keys it in manually. If the investigators have in some sense captured the data, they have not converted it to electronic form—it remains outside the study database and unavailable to study managers. Since few medical professionals leap at the chance to key in data, CRFs tend to accumulate in batches for weeks, waiting until somebody orders an unfortunate employee to key in data or the pile of CRFs justifies hiring a temp.

Handling data in batches makes perfect sense from the viewpoint of the investigational site because the data is available locally when needed. However, batches of unprocessed CRFs should make a very different impression on the program manager who is awaiting completion of a clinical study. Allowing important patient data to remain on paper deprives the study database of important information and ultimately risks delays in site close-out, database lock, and the delivery of information required for a regulatory filing. Handling CRFs in batches not only adds no value, but also wastes time and even commits what lean thinking regards as the ultimate sin: it reverses the value stream because delaying conversion of data to electronic form allows errors to proliferate. Both hand entering data on paper forms and keying in the hand-written data introduce errors because of legibility issues and careless mistakes. Even worse, while the CRFs wait in batches, the errors they contain are accumulating undetected. Nobody knows how many errors, what types, or in which data fields. Since data entry errors frequently occur in patterns indicating underlying problems, such as the design of the CRF or the training of the people who use it, allowing errors to linger undetected allows errors to proliferate. While data stays on paper, study managers have no way even to realize there is a problem, let alone recognize a pattern behind the errors, identify the cause, and take action to prevent recurrences. Meanwhile, site staff, also unaware that there is any problem, continue entering the same types of errors on additional CRFs during subsequent patient visits.

When site personnel finally key in the first batch of data and transmit it to the study database, study staff will identify numerous errors that could have been avoided by promptly keying in, reviewing, and validating data from early CRFs. Because of the needless proliferation of errors, the monitor or data manager responsible for validating the data must generate a correspondingly large number of queries. When the queries go back to the investigational site, they create more work for site personnel, who must dig out the original paper forms and compare the written entries to the values queried. These activities delay entry of correct data into the study database, further preventing study personnel from getting an accurate understanding of study progress. Moreover, the increased workload at the site makes it more difficult for site staff to keep up with the rest of their work, such as processing CRFs from subsequent patient visits, including keying in data. Thus, the study falls into a cycle of delayed data entry and needless proliferation of errors, queries, and detective work for query resolution.

The batches of accumulated, unkeyed CRFs represent exactly the kind of batch-and-queue problem that lean thinking seeks to eliminate. In the language of lean thinking, a query represents backflow. Filling out a CRF correctly to begin with eliminates the need to generate queries. Tolerating long periods of incorrect data entry because errors are going undetected is like allowing an improperly installed car part to remain in place until the end of the line, forcing additional staff to inspect, disassemble, and repair defective vehicles before shipment. In both cases, a flawed process needlessly wastes time, effort, and money.

In the case of a clinical study, the delays associated with something as simple as inefficient data capture can amount to weeks or months. The direct financial costs of additional labor to find and correct errors can be great, but the indirect costs of delayed site closeouts, regulatory filing, and market entry can sometimes amount to hundreds of millions of dollars. Inefficiency on such a scale can damage a drug's prospects and even jeopardize an entire development program.

Processing CRFs is not the only area where routine inefficiencies jeopardize clinical studies and drug candidates. Most of today's clinical trials still involve a great deal of variation in how studies are run between companies and even within the same company. Performance metrics are unavailable because standard practices do not require gathering the right data or analyzing it promptly or appropriately, or because the data necessary to generate performance metrics is hidden away in batches of unprocessed forms. Thus, managers lack information essential for managing studies more efficiently. At the end of the value stream, program managers wait, hoping for results that justify an early regulatory filing. Too often, study results do not justify seeking marketing approval. In other cases, studies produce the equivalent of last year's car model—a drug that reaches the market late, after delays that allow a competing product to establish a dominant position.

Match Technology with Tasks

Toyota did not owe its success to robotics. Indeed, Toyota's experience shows that inserting new technology such as robots into current processes does not automatically improve them. Many other attempts to use technology to optimize existing business processes have shown that inserting new technology may speed individual functions and yet fail to accelerate key processes appreciably. The true power of technology lies in enabling the redefinition of processes to be more efficient. Other carmakers who relied more heavily on robotics could not match the efficiency of Toyota's processes, which took advantage of technology only where it made sense. Toyota recognized that the value of technology lies in enabling process improvement, not embellishing existing processes. Experience in the drug industry confirms that the piecemeal application of technological enhancements to discrete portions of existing processes is unlikely to optimize anything. Inserting web-based EDC into existing processes has done little to shorten development timelines.

Following a revolution in computing and communications, clinical researchers can consider the use of an array of impressive technological tools. Such tools are ubiquitous, affordable, and in many cases already installed where needed. However, advances in computing and communications differ from most technological innovations by virtue of their versatility and flexibility. What a computer does depends on the software programmers write for it. What the internet and e-mail do depends on how information technology (IT) departments implement the systems that provide them, who is using those systems, and what they choose to communicate. Organizations can adapt such technologies as necessary to optimize almost any process. On the other hand, organizations can also fail to adapt computers and communications to specific tasks and processes. In those common cases, investments in technology bring few rewards.

Inefficiencies in clinical research have undoubtedly contributed to the disappointing numbers of new drugs approved in recent years. Many of these inefficiencies reflect the failure to reap the benefits of fully integrating new technologies into the work processes of clinical development. While most drug candidates fail because of lack of efficacy, clinical inefficiencies unnecessarily increase the time and cost of evaluating candidates and thereby reduce the number of candidates that can be evaluated. Despite technological enhancements here and there, the industry still conducts clinical studies using fundamental processes developed primarily in the 1940s, when the electromechanical calculator was king. Messages traveled on paper or by voice. Paper and file cabinets provided data storage. Physical locks and keys provided security. In the decades since A. Bradford Hill's watershed trial of streptomycin as a treatment for tuberculosis, communications and statistical techniques have made great strides. Improvements in data handling have simplified some aspects of clinical trials and greatly extended our ability to deal with massive amounts of data, far beyond anything Hill could have contemplated when planning studies in the late 1940s. The power of contemporary computers provides access to statistical techniques beyond the dreams of Hill and his colleagues. Today's researchers have witnessed the growth of computers from an expensive, unattainable curiosity to an indispensable tool of daily life in science, business, and the home. However, the existence of better technology has failed to produce commensurate gains in the efficiency of clinical research.

Clinical trials in the 21st century can take advantage of reliable tools that allow analyzing data as it becomes available during a trial and making decisions to improve efficiency. These tools can increase the efficiency of trials without lowering scientific standards or compromising the validity of conclusions. However, to reap the benefits of technological tools, it is vital to integrate them into the fundamental processes of clinical research as well as to optimize those processes. It is important to recognize that to accelerate clinical research to the full, the integration of technology must go far beyond the use of computers and communications to perform routine office work such as preparing budgets and memos and scheduling meetings. Chapter 9—"The Agile Platform"—describes the technological foundation necessary for putting adaptive research and agile clinical development into practice.

Objections to Adaptive Methods

While simple inertia contributes to slow adoption of information technology and data-driven management, the drug industry often cites three specific issues preventing the application in clinical research of the basic approach that has transformed other businesses. The issues cited are as follows: the need to ensure integrity and validity, the regulatory environment, and the sheer complexity of clinical studies. However, a thoughtful analysis shows that none of these issues poses an insurmountable obstacle to modernization.

Integrity and Validity

Study integrity and validity determine the accuracy of results. They are essential for any investigation. Much of the complexity of clinical trials derives from the need to ensure the accuracy of data. For example, about a third of study budgets pays for sending monitors into the field to ensure the accuracy of data recorded on study CRFs. Internal data management processes that identify and correct data problems further add to the cost of this fundamental process. These costs commonly reach millions of dollars for even modest-sized studies.

Ensuring study integrity, also called internal validity, requires accurate data as a starting point. It also requires following mandated processes (good clinical practices) and using statistical procedures to control for measurable biases such as confounding. Study validity denotes the ability to extrapolate study results to a larger population. A key consideration in validity is selecting study subjects that are reasonably representative of the target population.

In adaptive trials, sponsor and regulator alike want to ensure that any midcourse design changes take place without compromising study integrity and validity. The ability to make design changes sometimes creates discomfort in researchers accustomed to the traditional hands-off approach. The underlying concern is that making such changes requires making decisions too rapidly, increasing the risk of introducing unrecognized biases and errors.

However, sound adaptive designs provide a structured process that reduces the likelihood of introducing bias. Detailed prestudy analysis examines a variety of potential scenarios before defining rules, criteria, and procedures for deciding whether to make changes. In this sense, consideration of midcourse changes begins well before study inception; studies do not make changes "on the fly," but in strict conformity to criteria specified before the collection of any data. Planners of adaptive studies must devote considerable effort, including discussions with regulators, to ensuring integrity and validity. For example, if magnitude of the treatment effect is the basis of a sample-size reestimation, an outside group such as an independent data management committee might view the relevant data and decide whether to increase sample size in accordance with predetermined rules. Decision rules may also call for measures that make it difficult to infer the basis for a decision, such as stating ranges rather than precise values.

Rather than imposing an absolute and universal embargo on information about outcomes and patient assignments to different treatments, adaptive studies use techniques such as firewalls to control access to any information with the potential to introduce biases. Appropriate infrastructure for conducting adaptive studies allows continuous examination of trends affecting the quality of the information that will provide the basis for decisions (see Chapter 9). Furthermore, adaptive studies have certain advantages over conventional studies in addressing requirements for preserving integrity and validity. Adaptive studies often devote extra effort to ensuring the accuracy of the data and the correctness of operational procedures through earlier checkpoints and additional layers of internal checks. In many cases, adaptive studies allow greater time for designated parties to consider issues of validity and integrity precisely by allowing earlier access to some information. Adaptive studies and associated simulation tools may allow a more nuanced understanding of the relevant consequences of different decisions affecting integrity and validity. Finally, adaptive approaches also ultimately provide the flexibility to suspend activities while deliberating.

In considering whether adaptive studies adequately address issues of integrity and validity, it is important to consider common limitations of the comparator: the conventional study. The conventional approach can make it easy to overlook both flawed planning assumptions and inaccuracies in study data. Data is often less accurate in a conventional study because there is no opportunity to examine unusual or unexpected data during the course of a trial. For example, a subject who consistently has had about 10 grams of hemoglobin may unexpectedly register only 8 grams. This could represent a data error, perhaps altogether undetected because it falls within an acceptable range. It could reflect an unexpected effect of a test drug, a flawed operational procedure for collecting or recording data, or a failure to follow sound procedures. Because the conventional approach provides little or no opportunity to detect or analyze the basis for unexpected values, chances of identifying and correcting any underlying problems are slim. This limitation significantly impairs the ability to ensure data accuracy. In short, the conventional preference for keeping study management in the dark for the duration of a study does not necessarily ensure data accuracy or study integrity and validity.

The adaptive approach allows more options, but it also allows comparable or greater understanding and control of the issues affecting integrity and validity. As a result, adaptive studies can routinely manage issues affecting integrity and validity and uphold the same high standard as conventional studies.

The Regulatory Environment

While regulation has far-reaching effects on clinical research, the existence of regulations need not preclude the analysis and improvement of the processes involved in conducting clinical studies. Because both regulators and sponsors require credible results and therefore objectivity and reliability, the interests of regulators and sponsors largely coincide. Researchers require a solid, reliable basis for each decision point in the development process. Only reliable results from preceding steps can properly guide each subsequent step. Regulators also proceed by steps. In early studies, regulators focus primarily on assuring patient safety. In the large-scale pivotal studies that serve as the basis for marketing approval, regulators devote increasing attention to ensuring integrity and statistical reliability. However, throughout the clinical development process, both researchers and regulators are happy to see conclusive evidence for the efficacy and safety of a new drug. Researchers and regulators share many goals, such as exposing no more subjects to the experimental drug than necessary to achieve a reliable result and identifying any safety issues. Researchers and regulators alike should welcome any tools that contribute to meeting such common goals. Information technology and adaptive techniques increase the tools available, often allowing the acquisition of more nuanced information about new drugs.

The U.S. FDA and the European Medicines Agency (EMEA) acknowledge the importance of conducting clinical trials more efficiently. They have been receptive to methodologies that can improve efficiency without compromising validity and integrity. Properly designed and managed, adaptive methods meet these criteria. Chapter 7, "Planning Adaptive Programs," examines regulatory issues in greater detail.

The Complexity of Clinical Research

Does the sheer complexity of clinical research rule out the use of modern management techniques during studies? Studies increasingly involve substantial staff, large patient populations, and many sites, roles, data elements, and processes. There are always institutional review boards (IRBs) to consider and often independent data monitoring committees. Studies routinely operate across time zones, languages, and cultures. The need to make decisions that involve complex trade-offs adds another layer of complexity to clinical studies. For example, clinical decisions such as selecting an optimal dose during dose-finding studies often involve using experience and judgment to find an optimal balance of efficacy and safety. Weighing the need to exclude bias against the urgency of meeting timelines is not always a simple matter. In principle, an overzealous quest to exclude bias could consume resources on such a scale as to push costs beyond practical limits, leading to canceled studies—no results at all rather than results that are beyond any possible suggestion of inadvertent bias from sources known or unknown. Professional judgment must decide when enough is enough.

The volumes of information that clinical studies collect, validate, and analyze stagger the imagination—often hundreds of thousands or even millions of data points about thousands of patients, each of which must be traceable to its source. Even small studies involve many data points. Ensuring data accuracy adds to the complexity of clinical studies.

While the particulars of the complexity in clinical research are unique, its scale is not necessarily greater than the complexity that other industries routinely manage. People working in pharma may consider manufacturing simple by comparison. The natural assumption is that manufacturers repeatedly perform precisely the same steps to turn out precisely the same thing. People in pharma also tend to believe that everything in clinical research varies from study to study.

However, many activities, such as those involved in data capture and validation, are essentially the same in most studies. Furthermore, the view of manufacturing as a simple process is at odds with the reality of many modern manufacturing operations. The number of options in a modern car complicates management of the assembly process far beyond anything imagined by Henry Ford. Modern factories assemble cars on demand according to individual specifications, with optional engines, transmissions, braking systems, colors, interior trim levels, and, increasingly, electronic enhancements. Electronic features provide entertainment, navigation, climate control, and even automatic parallel parking. The number and complexity of electronic components in today's cars far surpass what is visible on the dashboard. Each car typically has multiple operating systems and even more software applications running in a variety of control units that are each responsible for the operation of multiple subsystems. These systems are sufficiently complex that more than 30% of the quality problems in a modern car relate to electronic and electrical systems.[13] Clinical research has no monopoly on complexity.

The complexity of clinical research does not exclude the use of modern management techniques—it demands the use of these techniques. Clearly, the efficiency of clinical studies depends on adopting such techniques. However, effective management methods affect quality as well as efficiency. Without efficient management based on timely information, it is much more difficult to ensure conformity to all scientific and regulatory standards throughout a study.

Conclusion

Techniques for adapting study designs in midcourse based on current study data hold the promise of greatly increasing the efficiency of clinical research. When an organization makes the decision to use such techniques, it should think in broader terms than learning to carry out a few types of discrete midcourse design changes. Since the same infrastructure for rapid data capture, validation, and analysis enables adapting study operations as well as study design parameters, there is every reason to use this infrastructure to support systematic operational adaptations based on current data and performance metrics. Applying the adaptive method to operations may provide even greater improvements in efficiency than adapting study designs.

Achieving the highest levels of efficiency in clinical research also requires making full use of integrated information technology, optimized processes, and modern management techniques. A key goal is to ensure that no effort, time, and resources go to waste. The commitment to adaptive research represents a major step toward achieving truly agile clinical development because it requires adopting infrastructure essential for the agile approach. Agile development goes farther, taking a more comprehensive, integrated, end-to-end approach than that associated with techniques for adapting study designs.

The next two chapters examine a variety of adaptive techniques that address issues in study design. Chapter 5 describes the many possible ways to adapt study operations based on a continuous stream of data and performance metrics. Chapter 6 shows the combined use of design adaptations and operational adaptations to improve the efficiency of an entire development program. The chapter also shows how the other aspects of agile development allow reaping maximum benefit from both types of adaptations.

References

1 Oxman MN, Levin MJ, Johnson GR, A vaccine to prevent herpes zoster and postherpetic neuralgia in older adults. NEJM. 2005;352(22):2271–84; also, supplementary appendix. Available from: http://content.nejm.org/cgi/data/352/22/2271/DC1/1.

2 Department of Veterans Affairs (US). Trial of varicella zoster vaccine for the prevention of herpes zoster and its complications. In: ClinicalTrials.gov [Internet]. Bethesda (MD): National Library of Medicine (US). Dec 29, 2000. [Cited Aug 12, 2008]. Available from: http://clinicaltrials.gov/ct2/show/NCT00007501.

3 Womack J, Jones D. Lean thinking. 1st Free Press Edition. New York: Simon & Schuster; 2003.

4 Taylor F. The principles of scientific management. New York: Harper & Brothers; 1911.

5 Drucker P. The practice of management. New York: Harper & Row; 1954.

6 Drucker P. Landmarks of tomorrow: a report on the new 'post-modern' world. New York: Harper & Brothers; 1959.

7 Drucker P. The essential Drucker: The best of sixty years of Peter Drucker's essential writings on management. New York: HarperCollins; 2001. pp. 120–21.

8 CenterWatch Staff. An industry in evolution. Third Edition. Boston: Thomson CenterWatch; 2001. p. 204.

9 Surowiecki J. The wisdom of crowds. New York: Random House; 2005.

10 Surowiecki J. The open secret of success. The New Yorker. May 12, 2008.

11 Ohno T. Toyota seisan hoshiki (The Toyota production system). Tokyo: Daiyamondo-sha; 1978.

12 Womack J, Jones D. The machine that changed the world. 1st Harper Perennial edition. New York: HarperCollins; 1990.

13 Fachet R. Open telematic platforms. In Proceedings of Automotive Electronics, 2006; The 2nd IEE Conference on Automotive Electronics. Mar 20–21, 2006;21–46.

— Chapter 3 —

Design Adaptations Part One: Finding the Right Dose

Design adaptations make studies more efficient or productive by assessing and adapting elements such as study size, doses, and patient-allocation ratios while a study is in progress. In most cases, design adaptations respond to information collected during the study itself. However, studies sometimes respond to data from other studies and a variety of other sources, including competitive business information.

The idea of allowing midcourse changes in clinical studies is not new. The statistical community and regulatory authorities have long accepted the legitimacy of interim analysis to test for early success or futility or to adjust sample size. Recent years have seen the number and variety of potential design changes increase and interest in using them grow. The FDA's Critical Path Initiative notes the need to streamline clinical trials and the potential of learning trials.[1] The Agency has issued guidance on the use of Bayesian statistics, an important tool in some adaptive methods, in clinical trials of new medical devices.[2] At the 2006 Conference on Adaptive Trial Design, the Agency announced plans for a series of guidance documents on adaptive methods. The FDA followed through in 2008 by publishing draft guidance on discussions following phase IIa trials, placing the topic of optimizing the next steps of development on the agenda.[3] The EMEA has also shown interest in adaptive methods, conducting workshops and issuing a reflection paper discussing possible restricted use of such methods in confirmatory trials.[4]

Regulatory agencies and the pharma industry are cooperating to promote wider understanding of adaptive methods and careful consideration of their

The Agile Approach to Adaptive Research, by Michael J. Rosenberg use. The industry group PhRMA convened a Working Group on Adaptive Designs in Clinical Drug Development. A summary of the working group's observations appeared in 2005.[5] *The Journal of Biopharmaceutical Statistics* devoted a special issue to adaptive studies in the same year.[6]

Several trends have combined to increase interest in adaptive methods. Advances in data collection and management provide earlier availability of clean data. There have been notable advances in statistical methods, infrastructure, and regulatory receptiveness. Later chapters address each of these areas in depth, but the reader may find brief comments helpful in the discussion of specific design adaptations in this and the following chapter. This chapter takes a pragmatic rather than theoretical or doctrinaire view of statistical techniques. Chapter 8, "Statistics and Decision Making in Adaptive Research," retains a pragmatic focus but offers some background on differences between frequentist and Bayesian methods.

Infrastructure plays a critical role in enabling adaptive methods, particularly by ensuring delivery of timely, accurate data and performance metrics. Without rapid data capture and validation, the risk of making midcourse decisions based on outdated or erroneous information precludes the use of adaptive methods. Chapter 9, "The Agile Platform," describes the infrastructure that adaptive methods require.

Not surprisingly, regulators judge potential use of adaptive methods on a case-by-case basis. In general, regulators are more likely to look favorably on the use of adaptive methods in early trials. Regulators review and approve possible design adaptations in advance, generally accept the use of Bayesian statistics in learning phases, and, to date, strongly prefer frequentist statistics in confirmatory trials. For additional discussion of regulatory issues, see Chapter 7, "Planning Adaptive Programs."

Background

As technology and methodology improved, researchers began to explore designs for data-dependent trials. For example, Wald introduced sequential designs in the 1940s[7]; Armitage introduced group-sequential designs beginning in the 1950s,[8] and Pocock and others provided notable advances in the 1970s.[9] Designs for response-adaptive randomization appeared in the 1970s with the work of Wei, Durham, Zelen, and others.[10,11] In the 1990s, Bauer and Köhne introduced a now widely used method for final data analysis that combines statistical tests on data collected before an interim analysis with tests on data collected afterward.[12] Today there is a growing range of increasingly versatile Bayesian designs. These designs continuously update outcome estimates as each new piece of information becomes available; Bayesian techniques for dose finding deserve particular note.[13]

It is important to recognize that many of the types of design adaptations described in this and the next chapter are not radical departures. Rather, they are descendants and variants of techniques developed over several decades.

Types of Design Adaptations

As an emerging field, adaptive research lacks a settled vocabulary. This can complicate the discussion of adaptive methods. For example, discussions about group-sequential and adaptive methods sometimes seem to imply that they are mutually exclusive. Some observers seem to consider the two different approaches as segments of the same continuum. Still other observers consider group-sequential methods as a particular subset of adaptive methods. Further complications arise when discussions seem to classify group-sequential designs that allow sample-size reestimation as adaptive but not group-sequential designs allowing early termination for futility or efficacy.

This book defines design adaptations to include any approach that may change some aspect of study design while the study is underway, regardless of the statistical methods, organizational structures, and operational procedures used to determine when, whether, and how to make such changes. On this classification, sequential and group-sequential methods rank as well-established adaptive methods rather than nonadaptive alternatives. From this viewpoint, sequential methods are an adaptive approach characterized by restrictions on the number of interim looks at study data. Sequential trials that allow early termination are adaptive, allowing a particularly drastic change to study design.

With this perspective, the debate about the merits of group-sequential techniques versus adaptive techniques becomes a comparison of the merits of different design-adaptive techniques for the purpose at hand. Group-sequential methods may offer less flexibility than some other adaptive methods. However, in some instances, group-sequential methods may also provide greater efficiency. For example, Jennison and Turnbull argue that a group-sequential design using an error-spending test can provide greater efficiency while achieving similar statistical power and comparable sample-size reestimates to those provided by adaptive techniques.[14]

However, other adaptive methods allow greater flexibility in response to the data that accumulates during a trial. The group-sequential approach is more rigid in the timing of changes allowed and in requiring specification of an error-spending function. Assessing the relative trade-off between flexibility and efficiency is difficult since surprising developments in internal study data or new external information may occur in the course of any trial, confounding the assumptions. Should this occur, the potentially more efficient group-sequential technique might not provide the flexibility required to respond appropriately.

Regardless of the adaptive techniques employed, it is best to specify any design changes and the criteria for making changes in advance. Adaptive trials do not allow making whatever changes may suddenly look desirable at any time during or after the trial. Plans for trials that adapt study designs must specify what can change, the criteria for making any change, and the parties responsible for deciding whether to make changes. Plans must also consider more scenarios and identify appropriate responses for each.

Most adaptive studies, including those described in this and the next chapter, change a single aspect of study design. However, a single study can employ multiple adaptive techniques. Furthermore, the development program for one drug can employ different techniques in different phases of development.

Order of Discussion

The following discussion of design adaptations roughly traces the chronological order of clinical studies from early safety testing through the confirmatory phase. The balance of this chapter first covers adaptive safety testing and dose finding and then turns to adaptive dose selection or pruning. Chapter 4 discusses sample size reestimation, seamless studies, adaptive randomization, and a variety of other adaptations.

Dosing Nomenclature

Dosing trials have two basic purposes. The first is finding the safe dose, which is somewhere beneath the maximum tolerated dose (MTD). The second is finding the optimal dose for subsequent testing, balancing both safety and efficacy. Traditionally, separate trials have fulfilled these two purposes for each drug. The earliest studies of safety use healthy volunteers unless exposing them to the test drug would violate ethical principles, as is true of many oncology products. Early studies using health volunteers usually provide no information about efficacy in the target population. However, the line between initial safety testing and testing that examines efficacy is blurring. Sponsors are often anxious for an early indication of efficacy, however preliminary or tenuous. If early testing involves patients with the relevant medical condition rather than healthy subjects, testing increasingly includes efficacy assessments. Furthermore, it has become possible with some types of drugs to detect indirect indications of efficacy in healthy patients. For example, the extent of binding by receptor modulators in healthy subjects may shed light on efficacy in diseased patients.

Dosing trials also differ in how they group patients and select doses to administer. For example, many phase I studies begin with small cohorts, often consisting of three subjects. Many dosing trials start with an extremely low dose and gradually escalate. Other dosing trials start closer to the expected range of efficacy but are prepared to reduce the dose. Phase II dosing trials typically group patients in treatment arms, with each arm receiving a different, predetermined dose. These trials try to choose the most promising dose among those tested. This approach works well subject to an important qualification that trials do not always meet: the doses selected for testing must include the optimal dose.

The limitations of conventional methods in phase I dose-escalation and phase II efficacy and dose-finding trials likely account for the failure of many drug candidates in late-stage trials. Limitations of methods used in these early phases can even contribute to problems that become apparent only after some drugs reach the market.

The terms used to describe these early studies can be confusing. Similar studies go by a variety of designations, including dose-escalation studies, dose-ascending studies, dose-finding-studies, dose-ranging studies, and phase I and phase II studies. Generally, dose-escalation studies focus on determining how well subjects tolerate a drug. Dose-finding and dose-ranging studies sometimes address safety alone but can sometimes involve testing both safety and efficacy. The following discussion will try to be clear about the objectives of each type of study.

Determining Maximum Safe Dose

Single Arm

What can change: Number of subjects used at each step of dose escalation, number of doses administered

Criteria for change: Number of subjects experiencing dose-limiting toxicity (DLT), with possible considerations of efficacy

Phase I studies generally provide information concerning safety, pharmacokinetics, and pharmacodynamics. The primary goal is to find the highest acceptable level of toxicity. A phase I study typically starts with low doses and escalates until the process establishes dose-limiting toxicity. For example, the standard dose-escalation design in oncology studies involves the 3+3 method, with cohorts of three patients. Phase I studies involving other indications often use larger cohorts.[15]

The 3+3 approach treats the first cohort at a very low dose. If no DLT occurs at a dosing level, a set of rules determines the next higher dose for the next cohort. If there are two or more instances of DLT, the dose for the next cohort reverts to the previous level. If one person experiences DLT, an additional cohort of three receives the same dose. With such expanded cohorts, doses increase as before unless two or more subjects out of six experience unacceptable toxicity. This defines DLT. The next lower dose represents the MTD. Another conventional dose-finding method uses cohorts of four healthy volunteers rather than three, with each cohort receiving a succession of three predefined, rising doses of the test drug and placebo. The lowest dose in each cohort is equal to the highest dose in the previous cohort.[16]

Interestingly, the 3+3 approach is further evidence that adaptive methods do not represent a radical departure from conventional practice. The 3+3 approach is itself adaptive—it determines the next dose based on patient-response data collected during the trial. However, the 3+3 approach has significant limitations. Dosing decisions consider only the response data on the latest cohort treated, ignoring data collected on response of previous cohorts. Restricting use of information to that on the last cohort increases the likelihood of inaccurately defining MTD. It is not rare for the 3+3 approach to identify an MTD that in later testing proves too toxic, requiring a step back in the development process to reassess toxicity. The 3+3 method also focuses exclusively on finding the highest dose with acceptable toxicity. Critics of the 3+3 approach attribute its common usage to familiarity and FDA encouragement rather than superior performance.[17]

In contrast to the standard 3+3 method, some adaptive dose-finding methods determine the next dose based on the cumulative body of information on all patients treated. Some adaptive methods for phase I studies seek to determine a dose with a combination of high efficacy and acceptable toxicity. Researchers often use these methods on diseased populations in oncology and other fields. Phase I studies may also seek to determine a dose with acceptable toxicity when the test drug is used in combination with different doses of an accompanying treatment.

Adaptive dose-finding methods often start with a dose believed to be both safe and reasonably close to where prior information suggests the final dose is likely to be. Studies may begin with a single cohort. After incorporating data on the response of each patient, the study can step the dose either up or down. This flexibility allows bracketing a target value and zeroing in with each new cohort. Alternatively, some adaptive approaches start by exposing small cohorts to different doses in order to define the dose-response curve and then zero in on the area of greatest interest (Figure 3-1). The goal is not just to identify a single MTD, but to define the safety/dose-response curve in the range of therapeutic interest.

Such adaptive dose-finding methods offer a more nuanced understanding of the dose-response curve and yield more information about the therapeutic range. Adaptive dose-finding methods also generally reduce costs and timelines by requiring fewer dosing cycles. Some methods provide for successive increases in the number of subjects in each group as the therapeutic range narrows. Data on the additional patients may increase understanding of the dose-response relationship in the range of greatest interest. However, the amount of information acquired depends on the method and its specific implementation. A more conservative approach starts with lower doses. This approach requires more cycles than some adaptive methods but provides greater safety while still taking fewer cycles than conventional methods, providing a more nuanced picture of dose response, and exposing fewer patients to noninformative doses.

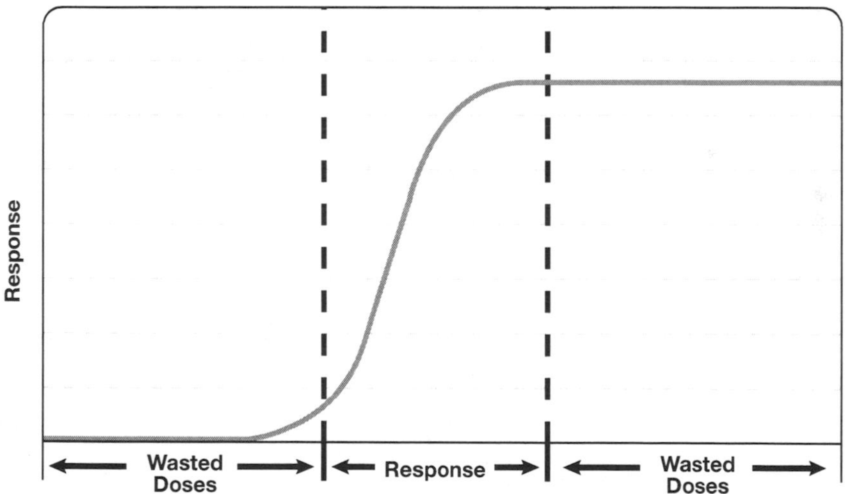

Figure 3-1. Identifying the therapeutic range. Adaptive dose finding seeks to minimize the number of noninformative doses by starting evaluation on the low side of expected toxicity, then adjusting doses up or down with each subsequent cohort to define a dose-response curve.

Conducting an adaptive dose-finding study requires the ability to monitor data as it is collected and make decisions about individual doses faster than with conventional methods. Continually monitoring data and making decisions more quickly present challenges. Among these is determining how much data provides a sound basis for a decision. There is always a delicate balance between having enough data to support a correct decision, waiting and accumulating more information than necessary, and acting based on less data with a greater risk of selecting a suboptimal dose. While there are formal techniques to aid decision making, choosing an adaptive approach to dose finding does not obviate the need for judgment; rather, adaptive methods seek to provide data earlier in the process, using each new result to build on the prior body of knowledge. This may provide earlier insights in the course of accumulating enough knowledge to justify a decision.

Like adaptive studies, conventional dose-finding trials also confront the challenge of determining how much information is enough. However, conventional trials generally provide less data and allow fewer decisions with fewer options.

Continual Reassessment Method

A leading technique for adaptive dose finding is the continual reassessment method (CRM), introduced by O'Quigley, Pepe, and Fisher in 1990.[18] This technique offers significant advantages over standard progressions that start at the lowest dose and move upward one step at a time. The CRM approach offers greater flexibility and the potential for gaining more knowledge about the test drug and gaining it faster. This includes identifying DLT and optimal or near-optimal doses earlier. As with the standard approach, CRM assumes that the highest tolerated dose is likely to be the most efficacious in later testing.

CRM can greatly improve efficiency in phase I studies focused on determining the DLT for a non-life-threatening disease. It can also be useful in studies that are attempting to determine efficacy as well as toxicity, including studies of oncology drugs that involve diseased patients rather than healthy volunteers.

Most CRM methods rely on a Bayesian statistical approach. CRM studies start by identifying a desired DLT rate and seek to find the dose most consistent with this rate. Using the best available information, often data from animal studies suggesting a dose-response relationship, a CRM study generates an initial estimate of the shape of the dose-response curve. CRM studies treat subjects one at a time. The CRM method includes the outcome for the most recently treated subject in estimating the optimal dose for the next subject. Like conventional designs, the CRM approach regards the definition of DLT as a binary (yes/no) event and assumes that the higher the dose, the higher the probability of toxicity.

The solid line in Figure 3-2 shows an estimated dose-response curve that might serve as the starting point for a CRM study. This curve is typical in suggesting a very low probability of DLT at the lowest dose. The curve estimates that, at dose level 4, 40% of patients would experience a DLT. The study could begin by administering this dose.

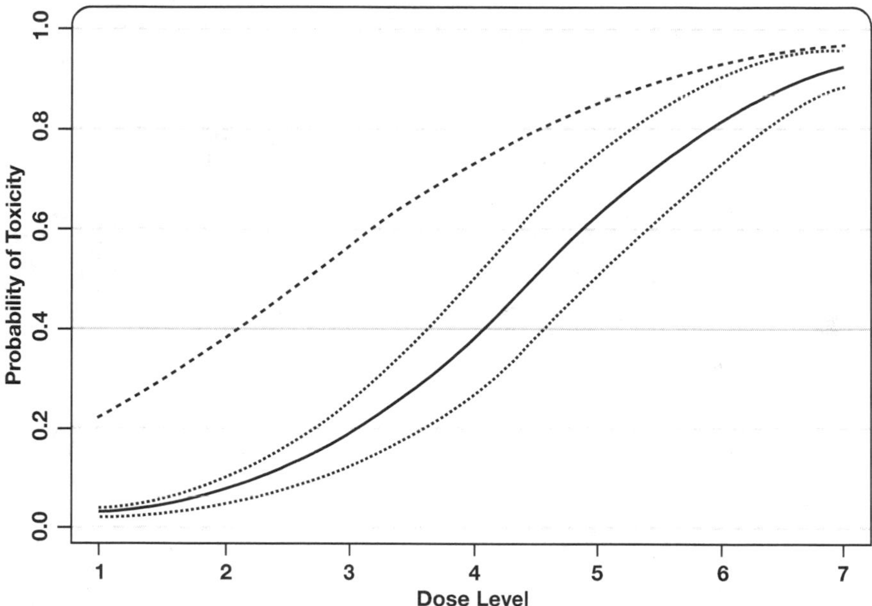

Figure 3-2. Dose-toxicity curves. The solid line represents a best estimate of the dose-response relationship before the study begins. This curve indicates that DLT is likely above dose 4. The study administers dose 4 to the first patient. A Bayesian statistical approach adjusts the dose-response curve after incorporating data on each patient's response (dashed line) and selects the dose for the next patient. This procedure repeats until a dose-response curve has minimal change. Variants of CRM provide a variety of ways to determine the seven dosing levels.

Source: Garrett-Mayer 2008.[19]

The two dotted lines indicate how the curve might move after incorporating data on the outcome for the first patient. If there were no DLT, the curve would move slightly to the right of the starting point; if there were a DLT, the curve would move slightly to the left. The study terminates either after treatment of a prespecified number of subjects or when the magnitude of incremental change after treatment of each subject falls below a designated level (say, <10%).

Variants of the Continual Reassessment Method

Over time, refinements to the CRM approach have addressed concerns about issues such as starting with a higher dose than conventional methods and using mathematical models that allow faster dose escalation.[19,20] Researchers can adjust the CRM method to consider the properties of the test drug and satisfy their safety concerns and preferences. For example, the approach can start with a lower dose or reduce the target level of toxicity. Some variants of the CRM approach incorporate aspects of the conventional stepped escalation and CRM methods. One variant starts with a very low dose like the conventional 3+3 method and uses a conventional 3+3 dosing cohort, or perhaps a 2+2 cohort. This variant escalates the dose gradually and switches to a CRM approach with the occurrence of the first DLT.[21]

Piantadosi proposes a method that starts by estimating 10% and 90% toxicity levels. The estimated dose-toxicity curve includes both of these points and an identified target dose. The first cohort of three patients receives the target dose.[22] Assessment of these patients provides the basis for redrawing the dose-response curve. This process repeats, incorporating the response data on each dosing cohort, until the study meets a preselected criterion such as the target dose changing by <10%.

CRM methods can also start with a larger selection of dosing levels and can select intervals between levels in a variety of ways.[19] One approach sets intervals between doses based on a modified Fibonacci sequence of 2, 1.67, 1.5, 1.33, and so forth. With this sequence, if the initial dosing level is, say, 100 mg, subsequent dosing will be 2 × 100 = 200 mg, 1.67 × 200 = 330 mg, 1.5 × 330 = 500 mg, and so on. Other variants described by Garrett-Meyer select dosing intervals based on a logarithmic scale, or on whatever method investigators are accustomed to using when setting dosing intervals with the 3+3 method.

Simulation for a variety of levels of toxicity shows CRM to be a faster and safer means of defining toxicity.[23] Adjusting doses based on responses in small cohorts or single patients reduces the number of subjects exposed to each dosing level. Adjusting among a greater number of dose levels is also likely to reduce risks. Regulators are generally receptive to adaptive dose finding in early learning-phase trials.

Case Study 3-1: Adaptive dose finding with the CRM method

A dose-finding study of samarium-153 in pediatric osteosarcoma[24]

To determine a maximally tolerated dose of samarium-153, a targeted radioactive therapeutic agent, researchers treated patients starting at 1.0 mCi/kg. The researchers used the CRM method to escalate or deescalate dose based on patient response. They established a target DLT rate of 30% and defined primary toxicity as failure of adequate recovery to hematologic toxicity, especially depletion of platelets. The study examined blood counts weekly.

A cohort of two patients received the initial dose with no toxicities. Incorporating this data, calculations set the dose for the next cohort of two at 1.4 mCi/kg. Four patients received treatment at that level, with two toxicities. Incorporating this data, CRM set the next dose at 1.2 mCi/kg. A cohort of two patients received this dose. There was one toxicity. CRM then calculated a dose of 1.1 mCi/kg. Two patients received this dose and there were no toxicities. The CRM method calculated the next dose as 1.2 mCi/kg for a second time.

The study identified the hematologic toxicity as the only DLT. While noting that two patients had moderate pulmonary toxicities, one at a dose of 1.2 and one at a dose of 1.4 mCi/kg, the researchers attributed the pulmonary toxicities to tumors rather than the test drug. When the researchers presented a poster, this study had yet to reach final accrual. However, at that time, the researchers had concluded that it is safe to administer samarium-153 to patients previously treated with chemotherapy, with the expectation of rapid hematologic recovery.

Another adaptive dose-finding study used Goodman's variant of CRM. (Case Study 3-2).

Case Study 3-2: Adaptive dose finding with the Goodman-Azhurak-Piantadosi version of CRM[21]

A dose-finding study of imatinib with irradiation in pediatric brainstem and intracranial gliomas[25]

This study estimated the MTD of imatinib with irradiation in pediatric cases of brainstem gliomas and recurrent malignant intracranial gliomas. The population was stratified based on use of enzyme-inducing anticonvulsant drugs (EIACD). The study employed a modified version of CRM that begins like a standard 3+3 dose-finding study, escalating from a low starting dose through a range of prespecified dose levels. Dosing started at 200 mg/m^2 and escalated through doses of 265, 350, 465, 620, and 800 mg/m^2, with possible deescalation to doses of 150 and 100 mg/m^2. The study administered the drug for a maximum of 13 courses or 52 weeks.

In view of possible associations of intratumoral hemorrhage with concomitant administration of the test drug and irradiation, researchers changed the protocol. The revised protocol delayed administration of the drug until two weeks after irradiation and excluded patients with a history of prior hemorrhage. Before the protocol change, 24 patients received treatment. Three of the 6 patients with brainstem tumor experienced DLT while none of the 18 patients with recurrent glioma did. After the protocol change, 5 additional DLTs occurred. Of these, 3 were among the 16 patients with brainstem glioma and 2 were among 11 patients with recurrent glioma who were not receiving EIACDs. After the DLT monitoring period, there were 10 more cases of intratumoral hemorrhage.

Analysis established the MTD for patients with recurrent high-grade gliomas without EIACDs at 465 mg/m^2. Analysis did not establish an MTD with EIACDs because there were no DLTs at the highest planned dose, 800 mg/m^2. The researchers recommended conducting a phase II trial. Although they noted the possible increased risk of hemorrhages, they also pointed out the relatively high spontaneous incidence of hemorrhages in brainstem glioma.

Other Bayesian Dose-Finding Methods

CRM is not the only Bayesian method of dose finding. Others include approaches based on Bayesian decision theory that maximize a predefined gain function and update after each response. There are also D-Optimal designs that use formally defined criteria for optimality.[16] A method with perhaps a closer resemblance to CRM uses escalation with overdose control.[26] Case Study 4-4 in the section of the next chapter on seamless phase II/III trials describes a study that includes use of another Bayesian dose-finding approach, general adaptive dose allocation (GADA).[27] This approach uses a normal dynamic linear model that allows flexible allocation of patients to doses based on optimization criteria defined in the model.

It is possible to combine a phase I trial of safety with a phase II trial of efficacy. One study design achieved this goal by using Bayesian techniques to determine the dose for the next patient based on considerations of efficacy as well as toxicity. The underlying principle is to allow selection only of doses judged both safe and efficacious. Determination of the starting dose considered relative levels of concern about beginning with doses that were too high versus beginning with doses that were too low. (Case Study 3-3.)

Case Study 3-3: Adaptive dose-finding combining phase I safety and phase II efficacy studies

Trial of tissue plasminogen activator (tPA) as treatment for ischemic stroke in children[28]

This study was a test of tPA as an experimental treatment for childhood acute ischemic stroke. The Bayesian dose-finding approach determines the dose for each successive patient cohort based on incorporating the latest efficacy and toxicity response data. The study's biostatisticians created a model for trading off efficacy versus toxicity based on physician input during trial planning. The biostatisticians asked the physicians to specify equally desirable probabilities for efficacy and toxicity. The planning process established criteria that enabled physicians to determine a set of doses that would have both low enough toxicity and high enough efficacy.

Biostatisticians then defined a function to evaluate the trade-off between the probabilities of efficacy and toxicity for each dose and, based on these trade-offs, calculate a value for the desirability of each dose. The study updated data on toxicity and efficacy continually. Each cohort received what the model identified as the most desirable dose after incorporating the latest data at the time of administration. The trial was a combined phase I/phase II trial in that it addressed both the phase I goal of assessing toxicity and the phase II goal of assessing efficacy.

Determining Optimal Dose (Pruning)

Multiple Arms

What can change: Doses administered, allocation of patients to dosing arms

Criteria for change: Efficacy and safety of each dosing level, with focus on selection of most promising doses for next-phase studies

Conventional dose selection evaluates a small, fixed number of doses, each in a separate treatment group of uniform size. Phase II dose-selection studies attempt to demonstrate both efficacy and safety and identify the most promising doses for use in phase III confirmatory trials. Phase II proof-of-concept (PoC) studies attempt to provide information on efficacy that can serve as a basis for dose-selection studies.

The methodology of optimal-dose-selection trials is attracting great scrutiny because many products fail in this stage. Phase II trials are especially important for smaller companies. Since their survival may be riding on the outcome, there is great pressure to progress a drug into more formal large-scale testing. Thus, phase II trials often require striking a delicate balance between generating enough information to advance to late-phase trials and needlessly spending time and resources when the viability of the drug candidate has not been established. This dilemma makes phase II trials one of the most challenging parts of drug development.

In fortunate cases, early safety studies will provide initial information on efficacy, as described earlier in this chapter. A phase I adaptive dose-finding study will have tried a number of doses, established a dose-response curve, and identified the dosing range of interest by tracking efficacy outcomes in addition to safety issues. However, most phase I studies provide little or no information on efficacy. Researchers must supplement safety information from a phase I study by conducting an early-phase PoC study to establish evidence of efficacy along with some indication of safety. Often such a study provides the only foundation for establishing appropriate test dosages for the dose-selection study. Following the PoC study, the dose-selection study may bracket the most promising doses from the PoC study with higher and lower doses. Although planners usually size these studies to ensure statistical power sufficient to differentiate the efficacy of different dosing arms, having that level of statistical power for every dosing arm may be unnecessary.

Based on available safety and efficacy data from earlier studies, planners of phase II dose-selection studies identify a range of plausible doses. Conventional studies often involve three or four active treatment arms plus a comparator, whether placebo or accepted treatment. Each treatment arm usually includes fewer than 100 subjects per exposed group. Outcomes usually track hard endpoints, but surrogate endpoints offer increasing appeal, especially with respect to outcomes that require measurement over long periods, such as survival in oncology products. At the trial's conclusion, analysis of the results will ideally identify a single dose or a small number of doses as safe and effective enough to justify going forward with large, expensive late-stage trials.

Improvements over Conventional Approaches to Dose Finding

The conventional approach—testing several arms of equal size for the full duration of the study—often wastes substantial time, effort, and money. Drugs enter this phase with limited information, mostly on short-term safety. There is often no information from testing individuals suffering from the indication. When studies start with such limited knowledge, expecting them to succeed in defining an appropriate dose for large-scale final testing is optimistic if not wishful. Poor dose selection in phase II studies contributes significantly to the disturbingly high rate of failures in phase III. The direct cost of phase III studies often runs into millions of dollars. Too often, these expensive studies mark the unsuccessful conclusion of costly development programs that started with impressive basic science.

The high cost of carrying all arms of a phase II dose-finding trial for the full duration of a study usually limits the number of doses tested. This markedly increases the risk of failure in the current phase or a more costly failure in a subsequent study based on phase II results. Testing relatively few arms and doses limits the acquisition of knowledge about the test drug. It also increases the likelihood of selecting a dose for confirmatory trials that is not at the optimal therapeutic level. The industry is thus seeking more efficient dose-selection approaches that allow economical testing of more doses to improve chances of correctly identifying optimal doses for phase III trials.

Adaptive approaches to dose selection offer several improvements over the usual reliance on a few treatment arms of equal size and duration. The fundamental principle is to start with a greater number of arms, to monitor efficacy and safety outcomes continuously, and to winnow the larger number of initial doses by terminating clearly inferior arms as soon as the accumulating information warrants. This approach often allows quickly eliminating outliers and focusing resources to generate much more information about the most promising doses. Decision making is more dependent on the comparative performance of arms within the study, especially early on. Adaptive dose-selection studies often allocate patients to treatment arms dynamically, with more patients assigned to the most promising treatment arms, rather than maintaining initial allocation ratios to a fixed number of treatment arms. This has the advantage of increasing the amount of data collected on patients taking the doses that appear most promising.

Dose Selection in Practice

Suppose a conventional dose-finding study has informational goals that require testing three doses plus placebo for eight months. The study carries four arms of 80 patients each for the duration. If all-inclusive per-patient costs are assumed to be $3,000 for startup and $1,500 for each study month, the cost for this conventional trial would be $4.8 million.

Now compare a hypothetical adaptive dose-finding study with the same informational goals and the same requirement to test 80 patients per arm and gathering data for eight months. Once again, study planners decide to test four arms: three dosing arms plus placebo. However, the study will terminate the least promising arms early. Figure 3-3 illustrates a four-arm dose-selection trial with adaptive pruning. The adaptive approach shown would save $1.2 million by pruning one arm a quarter of the way into the study and another arm halfway through.

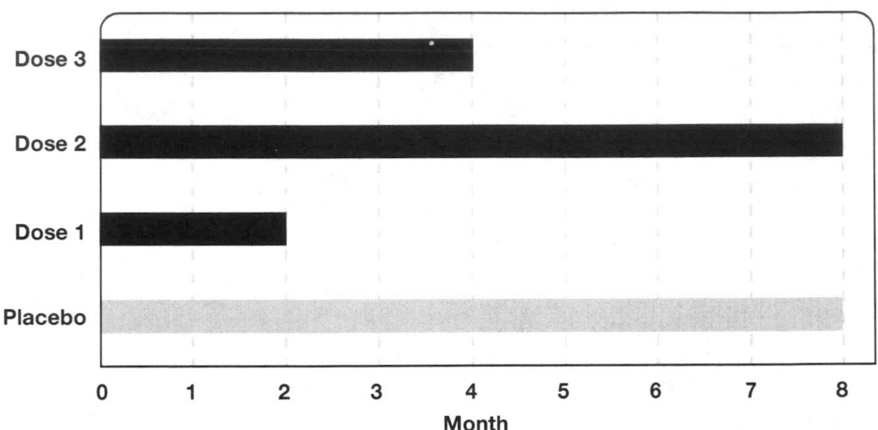

Figure 3-3. Four-arm adaptive dose-finding study comparing three dose levels of test drug with placebo. The study allows early discontinuation of two doses rather than carrying all arms for the full duration of the study.

Source: Health Decisions, Inc.

Suppose there is little knowledge about the dose-response curve in patients with the target disease. The sponsor recognizes the high risk of testing just three doses—there is no guarantee that any of the three doses falls in the optimal therapeutic range. Since the drug represents a huge opportunity, the sponsor places a premium on selecting the best dose possible, proceeding rapidly to a confirmatory trial and filing an early regulatory application. Based on earlier research, the sponsor feels confident that a large confirmatory trial will be justified when the dose-selection trial identifies an optimal dose. The sponsor wishes to test the drug at eight dosing levels against placebo in order to zero in on the most suitable dose for the confirmatory trial. However, the cost of a conventional nine-arm dose-finding trial based on the same costs would be prohibitive at $10.8 million.

An alternative dose-finding trial with adaptive pruning could test the desired eight doses against placebo for considerably less money because less promising arms are halted early. The design calls for pruning all but two dosing arms as soon as it becomes clear which two test doses offer the best balance of safety and efficacy (Figure 3-4). The sponsor would save $3.72 million as compared with a trial that carries all arms for eight months, reducing the total cost to $7.08 million.

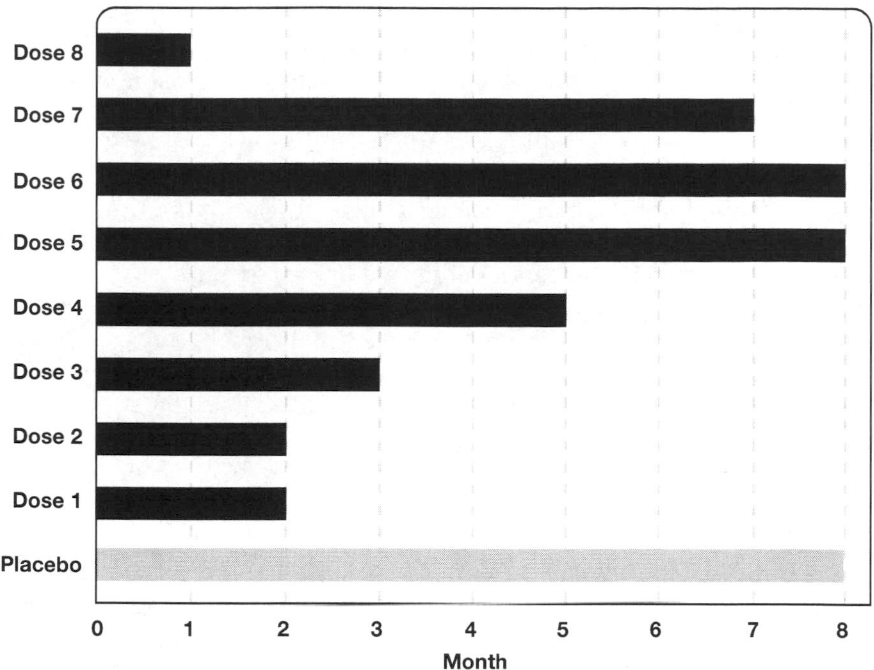

Figure 3-4. Nine-arm adaptive dose-finding study comparing eight dose levels of the test drug with placebo. However, the study administers only two doses plus placebo for the full eight-month period of the trial. Because the study tries eight doses of the test drug at smaller dosing intervals, it increases the likelihood of successfully identifying a dose with the best balance of safety and efficacy. Terminating six arms early limits the cost of testing additional doses.

Source: Health Decisions, Inc.

Optimizing Dose Selection

There are different approaches to deciding when to terminate arms early in dose-finding trials. Studies sometimes terminate arms following interim reviews performed at discrete, equal intervals. However, in the example shown in Figure 3-4, the timing of decisions to terminate arms depends on when information is sufficient to justify termination. In this example, the study drops three doses very quickly, two more by the halfway point, and one additional dose after five months of testing. Only three arms continue for the full eight months.

A more conventional four-arm study carrying all arms for the duration will have tested only three doses of the test drug rather than nine; unless fate smiles on the choices of the original three doses, there is a high likelihood of carrying forward one or two doses that fall outside the optimal therapeutic range. Assuming the same patient costs as above, the nine-arm design with early termination of some arms allows testing eight dosing levels for $7.08 million. The incremental cost of testing eight doses with adaptive pruning rather than three with conventional full-term arms is $2.28 million. This additional expenditure will prove to be an excellent investment if it increases the likelihood of choosing a dose with an optimal balance of safety and efficacy. That optimal dose is no guarantee, but it maximizes the chances of conducting a successful confirmatory study and winning regulatory approval. An adaptive dose-finding study may achieve more certain and useful knowledge about the most promising doses by rerandomizing patients from terminated arms. This provides an efficient way to gather data on a larger population exposed to the doses that patients are likely to receive in a follow-on trial.

Minimizing Costs Versus Maximizing Information

Sometimes the sponsor's highest priority may not be maximizing chances of selecting the most desirable dose for confirmatory testing. Because of financial constraints or uncertainty about the product's potential as compared to other candidates, the sponsor may be more interested in minimizing costs. The same adaptive approach can satisfy this requirement by emulating a conventional study that uses three test doses plus placebo. For example, an adaptive approach with four arms might terminate one test dose after two months and one after four months, completing the eight-month trial with the single most promising test dose and placebo. With these assumptions, the dose-finding trial would cost about $3.6 million. It would have tested the same number of doses as a conventional trial but saved one-fourth of the cost.

On all these dose-selection scenarios, the key trade-off is between overall cost and the quality of the information obtained. One useful way to evaluate this trade-off is to consider the cost per dose tested. Figure 3-5 shows that a four-armed study with adaptive pruning has lower cost per dose tested than a conventional nonadaptive study that tests the same number of arms. An adaptive study with a greater number of arms is most efficient, further reducing the cost per dose tested. Thus, the adaptive study with more arms may have higher absolute costs, but it produces superior dosing information for planning subsequent studies and provides the greatest efficiency. This is a powerful combination.

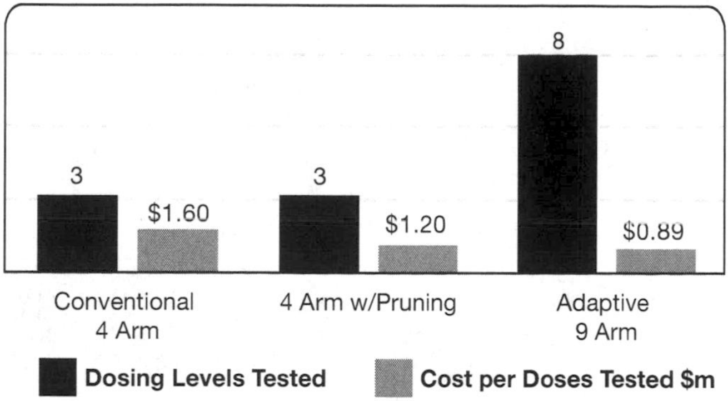

Figure 3-5. Adaptive dosing-finding studies can collect data on more dosing levels at lower cost per dose. The sponsor can choose to focus on maximizing the information gained while keeping costs reasonable, minimizing cost, or striking a balance between informational and budgetary requirements. Cost per dose tested is a measure of efficiency. The number of doses tested is likely indicative of the quality of the information generated.

Source: Health Decisions, Inc.

An important dimension not represented in Figure 3-5 is time to obtain information. While the three trials depicted have equal duration, adaptive methodologies can also sometimes obtain the desired information faster as well as at lower cost. Examining data earlier and more frequently means data for each patient can contribute to the information available to study managers. By contrast, a later one-time cross-sectional examination of the data at the end of the study may provide a less nuanced understanding of trial results, especially if the trial has tested fewer doses and thus gathered no data at all on some dosing ranges.

Surrogate Endpoints

Studies can use surrogate endpoints as outcomes without requiring changes in the adaptive procedures discussed above. One of the limitations with surrogates is that they are not the hard endpoints required for final testing in phase III. Rather, their utility rests on their correlation with an outcome acceptable to regulators. For example, studies that examine dosing in conditions with outcomes that take a long time to measure, such as multiple sclerosis or weight loss, often have shorter-term surrogates such as immune markers or short-term weight loss. These two examples, however, have very different correlation with long-term efficacy measures: experience suggests immune markers are often reasonably reliable indicators of long-term response, while short-term weight loss is not.

Certain modifications or combinations of the approaches outlined above can also enhance study efficiency during adaptive dose-ranging trials. For example, one phase IIb trial of a novel treatment for a chronic disease sought to include both standard care and placebo as comparators. This enabled simultaneously testing for superiority against placebo and inferiority against standard treatment. This effort included an initial 2-week period to compare four doses of the test drug, two active controls and placebo.[29] (See Figure 3-6.) After 2 weeks of treatment, an interim analysis provided enough information to drop two of the treatment arms using the test drug and one of the active controls. The study continued for 26 weeks, collecting data on the efficacy and safety of two doses of the test drug, the remaining active control, and the placebo.

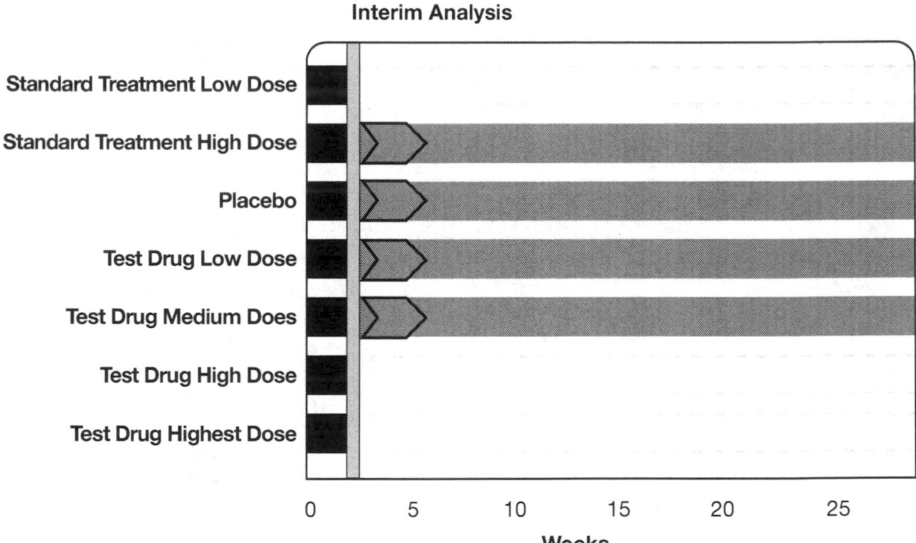

Figure 3-6. Rather than continuing all test arms for 28 weeks, this trial used a 2-week initial period to collect data on seven study arms and then, based on an interim analysis, stopped three arms and continued two arms of the test drug, one active comparator and placebo. At its conclusion, the study compared the most successful dose of the test drug with the active comparator for inferiority and with the placebo for superiority.

Source: Lawrence 2007.[29]

Bayesian adaptive methods have also proved useful in proof-of-concept studies with interim analyses to prune less effective doses or terminate the study for futility or failure to meet objectives. In one proof-of-concept trial, the Bayesian method used a normal dynamic linear model.[30] An advantage of this approach is generating probabilistic statements as a basis for pruning doses or, if the probability of demonstrating the desired level of efficacy is too low, as a basis for terminating the study.[31]

While adaptive dose finding has significant economic advantages, its greatest advantage is probably informational. Allowing a greater number of treatment arms with a greater range of doses spaced at smaller intervals increases the likelihood of identifying the therapeutic range with greater precision. The most notable benefits of this approach are to improve the outlook for the confirmatory trial that follows and to provide more nuanced information for regulators and prescribing physicians.

The adaptive approach to phase II dose-finding trials also carries another significant advantage—the possibility of seamless transition into phase III confirmatory trials. Provided the design and conduct of the phase II study conform to procedures and standards appropriate for a confirmatory study, phase II trials can carry the dosing arms selected directly into a confirmatory trial. Chapter 4 includes discussion of seamless designs that combine phases in this way.

Conclusion

Adaptive dose-finding techniques provide direct benefits in early phases, saving time and resources and often yielding more nuanced information about the test drug. However, the greatest benefits of adaptive dose finding become evident in confirmatory trials. By providing a better way to identify the optimal dose for late-stage testing, adaptive dose-finding methods reduce the chances of failure in the large, expensive trials that determine whether a drug merits filing for regulatory approval. Thus, adaptive dose finding can improve chances of avoiding the most disappointing outcome in clinical research—the failure of an entire development program.

Chapter 4 continues the examination of adaptive techniques, generally following the progression of clinical research from early studies through confirmatory stages. The focus now shifts from dose finding to sample-size reestimation, adaptive randomization, seamless combination studies, and other adaptive methods.

References

1 U.S. Department of Health and Human Services, Food and Drug Administration, Center for Drug Evaluation and Research (CDER). Washington (DC). Innovation or stagnation: Critical path opportunities report. Mar 2006. p. 12.

2 U.S. Department of Health and Human Services, Food and Drug Administration, Center for Devices and Radiological Health. Guidance for the use of Bayesian statistics in medi-

cal device clinical trials—Draft guidance for industry and FDA staff. Washington (DC). May 2006. Available from: http://www.fda.gov/cdrh/osb/guidance/1601.html.

3 U.S. Department of Health and Human Services, Food and Drug Administration, Center for Drug Evaluation and Research (CDER). Washington (DC). Guidance for industry end-of-phase 2A meetings. Sept 2008. Available from: http://www.fda.gov/cder/Guidance/8297dft.htm.

4 European Medicines Agency, Committee for Medicinal Products for Human Use. Reflection paper on methodological issues in confirmatory clinical trials with flexible design and analysis plan. London. Mar 2006. Available from: www.emea.europa.eu/pdfs/human/ewp/245902en.pdf.

5 Gallo P, Chuang-Stein C, Dragalin V, Gaydos B, Krams M, Pinheiro J. Adaptive designs in clinical drug development—an executive summary of the PhRMA Working Group. J Biopharm Stat. 2006;16:275–83.

6 Pong A, Luo Z, editors. Adaptive design in clinical research. J Biopharm Stat. 2005;15:535–752.

7 Wald A. Sequential analysis. New York: John Wiley & Son; 1948.

8 Armitage P. Sequential medical trials. Oxford: Blackwell Scientific Publications; 1961.

9 Pocock S. Group-sequential methods in the design and analysis of clinical trials. Biometrika. 1977;64:191–200.

10 Wei LJ, Durham SD. The randomized play-the-winner rule in medical trials. J Am Stat Assoc. 1978;73:840–43.

11 Zelen M. A new design for randomized clinical trials. NEJM. 1979;300:1242–45.

12 Bauer P, Köhne K. Evaluation of experiments with adaptive interim analyses. Biometrics. 1994;50:1029–41.

13 Berry DA, Müller P, Grieve AP, Smith M, Parke T, Blazek R, Mitchard N, Krams M. Adaptive Bayesian designs for dose-ranging drug trials. In: Gatsonis C, Kass RE, Carlin B, Carriquiry A, Gelman A, Verdinelli I, West M, editors. Case studies in Bayesian statistics V. New York: Springer-Verlag; 2001. pp. 99–181.

14 Jennison C, Turnbull BW. Efficient group-sequential designs when there are several effect sizes under consideration. Stat Med. 2006;25:917–32.

15 Ivanova A. Dose finding in oncology—nonparametric methods. Conventional or 3+3 design. In: Dose finding in drug development. Ting N, editor. New York: Springer Science + Business Media, Inc.; 2006. Chapter 4; p. 50.

16 Whitehead J, Patterson S, Webber D, Francis S. Easy-to-implement Bayesian methods for dose-escalation studies in healthy volunteers. Biostatistics. 2001;2:47–61.

17 Garret-Mayer E. Taking new agents to the clinic: phase I study design. Presented at: Neuroscience Institute, Medical University of South Carolina. c 2008 [cited Aug 12, 2008]. Available from: http://people.musc.edu/~elg26/talks/PhaseI.YukoClass2.pdf.

18 O'Quigley JO, Pepe M, Fisher L. Continual reassessment method: a practical design for phase I clinical trials in cancer. Biometrics. 1990;46:33–48.

19 Garrett-Mayer E. Understanding the continual reassessment method for dose finding studies: an overview for non-statisticians. Johns Hopkins University, Dept. of Biostatistics Working Papers. Working Paper 74. Berkeley Electronic Press [Internet]. Mar 2005 [cited Aug 12, 2008]. Available from: http://www.bepress.com/jhubiostat/paper74.

20 Garrett-Mayer E. The continual reassessment method for dose-finding studies: a tutorial. Clin Trials. 2006;3:57–71.

21 Goodman S, Zahurak M, Piantadosi S. Some practical improvements in the continual reassessment method for phase I studies. Stat Med. 1995;14:1149–61.

22 Piantadosi S, Liu G. Improved designs for phase I studies using pharmacokinetic measurements. Stat Med. Aug 15, 1996;15:1605–18.

23 Quigley J. Another look at two phase I clinical trial designs. Stat Med. 1999;18:2683–90; discussion 2691–2.

24 Loeb D, Garret-Mayer E, Sgouros G, Wharam M, Scott T, Schwartz C. A dose finding study of 153SM-EDTMP in patients with high risk of osteosarcoma. Poster at 12th Annual Meeting of Connective Tissue Oncology Society, Venice, Italy. Nov 2–4, 2006.

25 Pollack, I, et al. Phase I trial of imatinib in children with newly diagnosed brainstem and recurrent malignant gliomas: A Pediatric Brain Tumor Consortium report. Neuro Oncol 2007;9:145–60.

26 Tighiouart M, Rogatko A. Dose-escalation with overdose control. In: Chevret S, editor. Statistical methods for dose-finding experiments. New York: John Wiley & Sons; 2006. Chapter 8, pp. 173–88.

27 Krams M, Lees KR, Berry DA. The past is the future: innovative designs in acute stroke therapy trials. Stroke. 2005;36:1341–7.

28 Whelan H, Cook J, Amlie-Lefond C, Hovinga C, Chan A, Ichord R, deVeber G, Thall P. Practical model-based dose-finding in early phase clinical trials: optimizing tPA dose for treatment of ischemic stroke in children. University of Texas MD Anderson Cancer Center Year 2008 Working Paper 1. Collection of Biostatistics Research Archive, Berkeley Electronic Press [Internet]. Jan 2008 [cited Aug 12, 2008]. Available from: http://www.bepress.com/cgi/viewcontent.cgi?article=1040&context=mdandersonbiostat.

29 Lawrence D. Phase II/III adaptive design with treatment selection: a case study. Presented at: Seminar on Adaptive Designs in Drug Development. Basel Biometric Section, European Federation of Statisticians in the Pharmaceutical Industry. Jun 15, 2007. Basel. Available from: http://www.efspi.org/PDF/activities/international/adaptive_design_Basel_2007/7_Adaptive_Designs_Case_Study_3_DL.pdf.

30 Smith M, Jones I, Morris M, Grieve A, Tan K. Implementation of a Bayesian adaptive design in a proof-of-concept study. Pharm Stat. 2006;5:39–50.

31 Smith MK, Morris M, Jones I, Grieve A, Tan K. An adaptive design for dose-response using the normal dynamic linear model. Oral presentation at the thirteenth meeting of the Population Approach Group in Europe. June 17–18, 2004. Uppsala, Sweden. Available from: www.page-meeting.org/page/page2004/oral.pdf.

— Chapter 4 —

Design Adaptations Part Two: Additional Design Changes

Finding the doses of a new drug that appear to offer the best combination of safety and efficacy marks an important milestone, but not even the halfway point on the road to registration. The new drug must still undergo large-scale testing to provide a statistically significant assessment of the drug's efficacy for the target population. A range of techniques for adapting study designs may provide opportunities to accelerate late-stage development, reduce costs, or allow the acquisition of more comprehensive and nuanced information about the test drug. Such techniques include the design adaptations discussed in this chapter:

- Sample-size reestimation
- Seamless studies
- Adaptive randomization
- Other adaptations
  - Biomarker adaptive
  - Treatment switching
  - Adaptive hypothesis (e.g., noninferiority to superiority)

Sample-Size Reestimation

What can change: size of study population in one or more groups

Criteria for change: magnitude of treatment effect, magnitude of placebo response, acceptable levels of type 1 and type 2 error, rate of patient compliance, rate of patient dropout, covariate values, and variance of the outcome data

Sample size is the primary determinant of cost, duration, and complexity for individual studies and entire development programs. Testing more patients takes more money, time, and effort. This constitutes a powerful economic argument for identifying the smallest sample size that will produce definitive results. However, standard industry practice often selects sample sizes significantly greater than actual needs as a hedge against falling short of the statistical power required. For much of the history of clinical development, "overbuilding" has been the most rational response to a disturbing reality: accurately determining the required sample size in advance involves as much luck as science. The one drug in five that successfully completes phase III trials almost certainly has at least one overbuilt study in its development history.

The Trouble with Planning Estimates

When study planners determine the study size, the information needed for precise determination is simply unavailable. Determinants of sample size include:

- the effect size in the comparison group (either another drug or placebo);
- the magnitude of difference (δ) between that comparator and the product under evaluation;
- the statistical power to detect that difference ($1-\beta$, where β is the probability of mistakenly concluding that no difference exists when a difference actually does, a type 2 error);
- type 1 error (α), the chance of concluding that the two groups differ when in reality they do not, also affects considerations of sample size.

What statisticians aptly call nuisance parameters also influence determination of sample size. Nuisance parameters include:

- the variance of the outcome data (σ);
- the magnitude of the placebo effect;

- covariate values;
- nonstatistical elements such as dropout rate and patient compliance.

Among all these parameters, only α is known at the outset of the study, due to the tradition of setting $\alpha = 0.05$.

Planners may estimate the expected magnitude of treatment effect based on data from an earlier trial too small to support definitive conclusions. Other possibilities include using data from a somewhat similar trial of a drug in the same class or relying on the judgment of experienced practitioners. In many cases, the practitioners have little or no direct experience with the test drug. Some planning estimates consider information from a combination of such sources. Estimates of other planning parameters, such as rates of patient dropout and compliance, may rest on even weaker foundations.

Furthermore, even when planning estimates are accurate at study inception, external developments may force reassessment during the study. For example, new results from related studies may contradict the basis for earlier estimates or an outside body may revise the standard of treatment of the target disease, making a change in comparator advisable. In such cases, an accurate initial estimate of treatment effect may still yield a smaller than expected treatment difference or event rate. Thus, a study may fall short of the required statistical power for a wide variety of internal and external reasons.

The High Cost of "Underbuilt" Studies

Despite precautionary overbuilding, underbuilding remains a threat. If the estimated treatment effect renders a trial's sample size too small to yield a statistically significant outcome, the only corrective measure available at the end of a conventional trial is to conduct an entirely new study. While the first trial will contribute to better estimates of planning parameters for a second attempt, circumstances may raise doubts about the wisdom of making the large additional investment required. For example, the time required for a new trial may enable a competitor to bring a similar drug to market first. The sponsor must then revisit key assumptions in the business plan for the test drug. Reaching market second or third instead of first can reduce expected revenues by half or more. An additional trial increases development costs. Later market entry almost certainly increases marketing costs. The sponsor must reassess whether the test drug remains the best use of limited R&D and marketing funds—or whether the drug even remains viable. Writing off the cost of the entire trial and all preceding development may seem preferable to additional spending on a troubled program.

Misestimating sample size has human as well as economic consequences. Exceeding the required sample size needlessly exposes some patients to experimental treatments. Thus, for both economic and ethical reasons, the goal should be rightsizing each trial—exposing just the right number of patients to the new treatment to achieve the desired informational goals.

The Benefits of Reestimation and Rightsizing

Sample-size reestimation provides the opportunity for midcourse corrections based on replacing the estimated values used for planning with actual values observed during the trial. It is true that midcourse measurements may themselves differ from final values for key parameters and thus lead to erroneous estimates of sample size. Thus, the decision to use sample-size reestimation comes down to a judgment of the more reliable source of values for key parameters: whatever information was available at the planning stage or partial data from treatment of an actual sample of the target population with the right dose of the test drug. Experience suggests the latter is usually the better guide.

Multiple course corrections may sometimes be necessary to arrive at the desired informational goal with maximum efficiency. However, the first sample-size reestimation should usually take place after observed values are likely to have become reasonably stable. In most cases, this will be at least halfway through the study. Moreover, study planners and managers must devote careful attention to statistical techniques that ensure continued design integrity.

Besides allowing corrections to mistaken planning assumptions, sample-size reestimation can also allow studies to take advantage of other adaptive techniques without jeopardizing statistical power. For example, techniques for adaptive randomization, while offering potentially great benefits such as allocating a greater proportion of patients to the most promising treatments, may have the effect of increasing error rates. In that event, sample-size reestimation can increase study population to compensate.

The difficulty of producing a sample-size estimate borne out by actual trial data has inspired extensive research into different methods of adjusting sample size. A variety of methods is already in use.[1] The pharmaceutical industry's Adaptive Design Working Group recommends that study planners routinely consider use of sample-size reestimation.[1] If anything, the recommendation should be stronger: the presumption should be in favor of using sample-size reestimation absent a strong reason not to.

Reestimation and Trial Stages

Preserving statistical validity is a major goal of reestimating sample size. For multiple comparisons of an outcome measure (focusing on the magnitude of treatment effect, δ), it is important to consider repeated measures and preservation of type 1 error, α.[2] A number of accepted approaches involve using flexible alpha-spend functions at different stages of the study. A researcher can decide how to distribute a total α of 0.05, and some spending functions actually allow a total spend slightly greater. A very low alpha spend (say, 0.0001) early in the process effectively precludes a statistical basis for early termination, but it allows sample-size reestimation and a midstudy glimpse of study progress. The cost (alpha spend) in this case is very low, providing an almost "free" look because it does not reduce the final *p*-value required to achieve significance. However, a group firewalled from the study team must take responsibility for the midcourse look in order to maintain blinding, if present, and prevent possible introduction of inadvertent bias.

Sample-size reestimation plays an important role in two-stage study designs. At the conclusion of the first stage, a rule defined in the study protocol uses data gathered in the first stage to determine the appropriate sample size for the second.[3] Two-stage designs can condense timelines for dose-finding (phase II) and confirmatory (phase III) evaluations. Figure 4-1 illustrates a two-stage design.

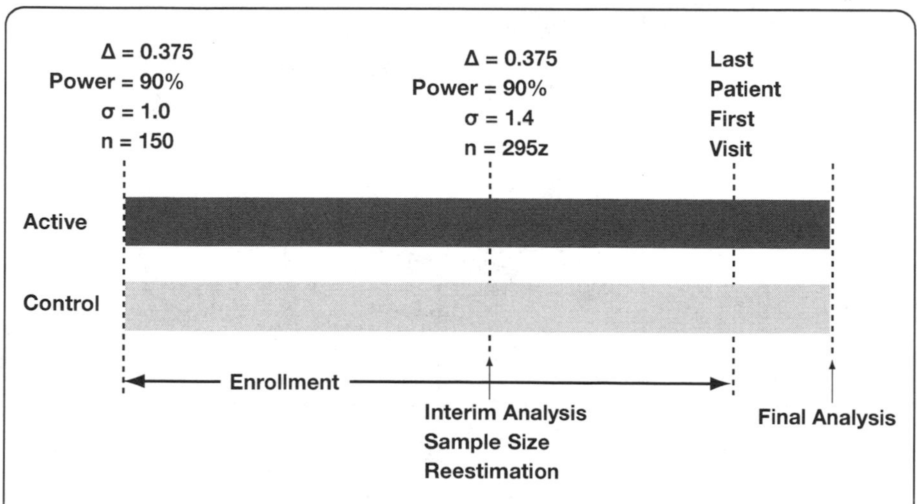

Figure 4-1. A two-stage design for sample-size reestimation. Without an increase in sample size, statistical power drops to 64%, far below required levels. Source: Thomas 2007.[4]

Rules to Restrict Reestimation

The rule for reestimating sample size may include restrictions to prevent undesirable outcomes. For example, a rule may limit the size of increases in order to keep costs within reasonable bounds. A rule may also restrict reestimation to increases. This type of sampling rule reflects a strategy that regards the initial sample-size estimate as the lower bound. Planners select the initial sample size from the lower range of estimated values in order to avoid unnecessary expense and reduce patient exposure to new treatments in the first stage of the study. If interim data dictates, an increase in sample size can still achieve the desired power and informational goals.

Adjusting Sample Size for Nuisance Parameters

As noted, factors other than magnitude of effect influence the determination of sample size. For example, the greater the variability of the data, the greater the number of subjects needed to demonstrate a significant effect. Figure 4-2 shows how even modest increases in variability can reduce study power markedly.

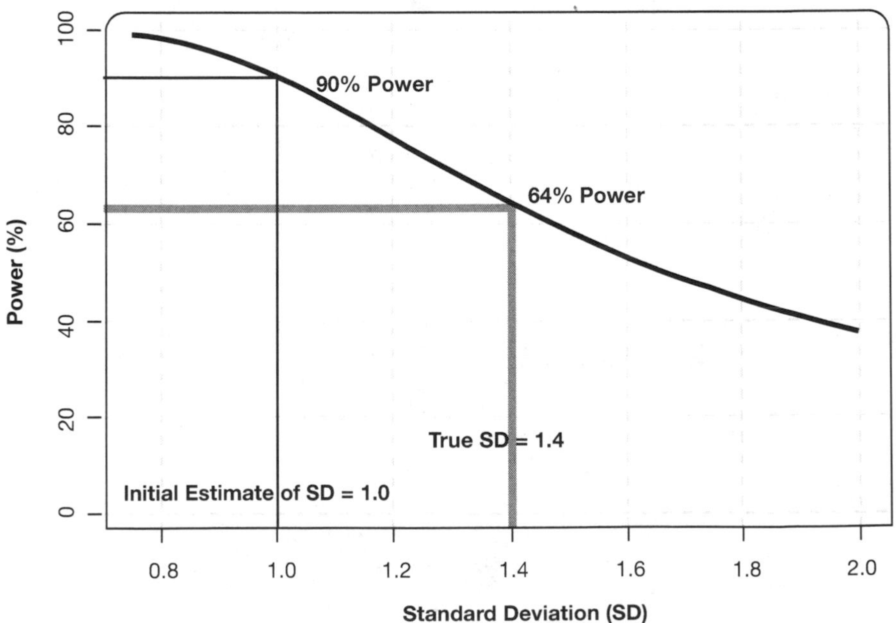

Figure 4-2. A study's statistical power, or the ability to detect a given magnitude of treatment effect, drops as the variability of data increases.

Source: Thomas 2007.[4]

Operational Considerations

Important operational questions include who is to perform sample-size reestimation based on nuisance parameters and whether data is to be blinded. While sample-size reestimation based on the observed treatment effect increases the likelihood of unblinding, reestimation based on nuisance parameters does not; it does not involve analyzing the magnitude of the treatment difference. As an operational convenience, in-house staff can perform reestimation based on nuisance parameters.[5] Nevertheless, this technique may still raise concerns about the possibility of introducing bias. For example, there may be some risk that, while accessing data on nuisance parameters, someone may gain inadvertent access to information about observed treatment effect. Such concerns may warrant having an external party review the data even for sample-size reestimation based on nuisance parameters. The type 1 error rate requires attention in sample-size reestimation. However, this issue is usually manageable, particularly when sample size increases.

Case Study 4-1 describes a psoriasis trial that adjusted sample size based on a nuisance parameter, in this case the magnitude of the placebo effect. The study plan provided for keeping sample size open, increasing as necessary until the standard error in the treatment difference was small enough to provide the statistical power desired.

Case Study 4-1: Trial of new therapeutic agent for treatment of psoriasis.

Upward adjusting sample-size reestimation with maximum information design based on uncertainty about magnitude of the placebo effect[6]

Planners of a study of a new therapeutic agent for the treatment of psoriasis were uncertain about the likely magnitude of the placebo effect and thus the magnitude of the treatment difference. The primary endpoint was measurement of the Psoriasis Area and Severity Index, PASI-75, at week 16.

The initial estimate of the placebo rate was 7.5%, with the likely range estimated at 5%–15%. The study required 95% power to detect a 10% improvement over treatment with placebo. The sponsor established the 10% improvement as a requirement to differentiate the drug from existing treatments. Thus, the study planners knew that this treatment difference defined the standard of success. The planners could only estimate the magnitude of the placebo effect that the study would actually observe. To ensure maintaining adequate statistical power to detect a 10% difference in treatment effect between the test drug and placebo despite the uncertainty about the magnitude of the placebo effect, the plan used a maximum information design. With this design, the standard error had to be low enough to detect the 10% treatment difference with the required 95% power. Using data collected during the trial, the study reestimated the sample size to the level required to reduce the standard error in the treatment difference enough to ensure adequate statistical power.

Adjusting Sample Size for Observed Treatment Effect

Because repeated measures of the same outcome are more likely to produce a positive result, an interim sample-size reestimation requires attention to alpha- and beta-spend considerations—statistical measures to prevent reaching faulty conclusions. The first sample-size reestimation takes place after accumulating enough data to assure stable effect estimates but with enough time to implement any changes that may result. Plans usually call for performing the first sample-size reestimation when the study has collected about half of the information expected. The study plan should limit the purpose of re-estimating sample size to achieving prespecified statistical goals. Setting the alpha-spend function very low rules out having a basis at the interim review for early stopping for futility or success. The focus of the review is entirely on a midcourse reality check of the initial estimate of the magnitude of effect.

In a recent oncology study, sample-size reestimation allowed the study to conclude nine months earlier than estimated in the original plan. An interim analysis demonstrated a much greater effect size (δ) than anticipated. The savings from the resulting sample-size reduction included the cost of additional recruitment, supplies, treatment, monitoring, and follow-up for patients in excess of the necessary sample size. All told, sample-size reestimation led to savings of more than $16 million. Furthermore, concluding the study nine months earlier enabled the test drug to reach market and begin generating revenues that much sooner (Health Decisions, Inc.).

Case Study 4-2: Sample-size reestimation: the A-HeFT trial of Bidil as a treatment of heart failure in African Americans

Sample-size reestimation based on observed treatment difference[7]

The A-HeFT study compared the safety and efficacy of Bidil with placebo in treating stable symptomatic heart failure in black patients already receiving standard treatment for the condition. Patients received tablets of the drug that is a combination of isosorbide dinitrate and hydralazine. Daily target doses were 120 mg of isosorbide dinitrate and 225 mg of hydralazine. The study's primary endpoint was a composite score based on all-cause mortality, first hospitalization for heart failure, and change at six months in a quality-of-life measure versus baseline. Based on data from prior studies, planners designed the A-HeFT trial to detect a treatment difference equivalent to 22.8% of a standard deviation with 80% power in a sample size of 600 patients in two arms.

The second of two interim analyses performed the SSRE. The study scheduled the second interim analysis when half of the 600 patients had completed six months of follow-up. The study reestimated effect size based on the observed mean difference in composite scores for the two arms divided by its standard deviation. The reestimation established that for $\alpha = 0.05$ study population would have to increase to 900. However, the FDA advised using $\alpha = 0.02$ for sample-size reestimation. This increased the required sample size to 1100. The researchers stopped the trial early, after randomization of 1014 patients. Analysis showed that the test drug provided a statistically significant benefit in mortality, necessitating discontinuing placebo treatment of the control group for ethical reasons.

Case Study 4-3 illustrates sample-size reestimation based on greater than expected variability in a key measure—in this case, treatment effect. This case study shows the value of sample-size reestimation but also provides a vivid example of the degree to which design adaptations are dependent on operational efficiency and infrastructure. The use of SSRE did allow substantially reducing sample size in the study described. However, flawed operational processes and infrastructure wiped out almost half of the benefit. Infrastructure must provide not only a basis for timely decisions but also the means to communicate and execute decisions quickly.

As shown in Case Study 4-3, adaptive randomization requires an efficient, centralized mechanism that can not only randomize patients quickly, based on the latest information, but also halt randomization immediately when the study has enrolled the desired number. The lack of such a mechanism prevented this study from reaping the full benefit of sample-size reestimation. Chapter 5, "Operational Adaptations," describes techniques for ensuring that study operations function at a high enough level to enable design adaptations. Chapter 9, "The Agile Platform," addresses infrastructure requirements.

Case Study 4-3: Sample-size reestimation in a trial of lumiracoxib versus ibuprofen in treatment of hypertension in patients with osteoarthritis and controlled hypertension

Reestimation based on variability of treatment effect[8]

This study sought to determine for its target population whether 100 mg of lumiracoxib once daily would have as great an effect on blood pressure as 600 mg of ibuprofen taken three times daily. The study established a primary outcome measure of change in 24-hour mean systolic ambulatory blood pressure from baseline to week 4.

Planners set an initial sample size of 1,020 patients in two equal arms based on an estimate of the standard deviation for the primary endpoint as 11 mmHg. After 600 patients completed the study, a blinded interim review found that the standard deviation observed in the study was only 8.33 mmHg. This allowed detecting a difference of 2 mmHg with a sample of 548 patients at 80% power and 5% significance.

Reducing sample size to 548 patients would have allowed greatly reducing study costs. However, the study had already randomized 787 patients by the time the decision to reduce sample size had been made and communicated. Thus, inefficient study operations cut potential savings from sample-size reestimation in half. The original sample size would have enrolled 472 patients more than necessary, but the study still enrolled an excess of 239 patients.

Testing did observe that blood pressure in patients taking lumiracoxib decreased while blood pressure in patients taking ibuprofen increased. Study data yielded an estimated difference in pressure of 5.00 mmHg with a 95% confidence interval on values for lumiracoxib of −6.1 mmHg to −3.8 relative to values for ibuprofen.

In another large trial, researchers tested azithromycin as a treatment for atherosclerosis and related disorders (Case Study 4-4). In this case, external information provided by the trial's independent data management committee was the impetus for reconsidering the original determination of sample size. In the committee's view, a reduction in the incidence of primary events smaller than the reduction used in planning the trial would still have clinical significance. The study increased sample size to allow detecting a smaller difference in event rate. The study enrolled 7,747 patients and reached a statistically significant finding. However, that finding was that azithromycin failed to provide the desired benefit.

Case Study 4-4: Sample-size reestimation: the WIZARD trial of azithromycin as a treatment of atherosclerosis

Reestimation based on external information about magnitude of clinically significant difference in event rate[9]

The Weekly Intervention with Zithromax for Atherosclerosis and Its Related Disorders (WIZARD) investigated the efficacy of azithromycin (Pfizer's Zithromax) in treatment of atherosclerosis. Evidence suggested that atherosclerosis may be an inflammatory disease, that infectious microorganisms may play a role, and that *Chlamydia pneumoniae* may be among these microorganisms. Therefore, researchers decided to test whether an antichlamydial antibiotic could slow the progression of coronary heart disease. The randomized, placebo-controlled WIZARD study administered a 3-month course of azithromycin compared with placebo. The primary endpoint was a composite of time to a recurrence of myocardial infarction, death, a revascularization procedure, or hospitalization for angina. The study plan called for enrolling 3,300 patients based on an initial estimate of the expected event rate.

However, based on information that became available after the start of the trial, the independent data management committee advised that a smaller reduction in event rate than the planning estimate would still be clinically significant. The study increased sample size in order to detect the lower difference in event rate with the desired statistical power. The study enrolled 7,747 test patients and randomized 3,879 to the azithromycin treatment arm and 3,868 to placebo. After a median of 14 months of follow-up, the study found no significant reduction in the likelihood of a primary event with azithromycin versus placebo.

Finally, it is worth noting the possibility of studies that provide for early stopping as well as sample-size reestimation.

Seamless Designs: Combining Multiple Phases

What can change: conventional separation of different trial functions into phases, elimination of between-phase pauses, focus of testing

Criteria for change: prespecified conditions for advancing to the next phase of development (e.g., from safety assessment to efficacy testing or dose selection to confirmatory testing)

Between-phase pauses have played an important role in drug development, allowing for a period of analysis, reflection, planning, and discussions with regulators. These pauses were essential when all data became available only at the very end of each study. However, recently developed tools for rapid data capture, communication, cleaning, and analysis open new possibilities. New data from anywhere in the world can reach a study database almost immediately. Database lock can take place rapidly, perhaps on the same day as the last patient visit. Such capabilities raise serious questions about whether conventional delays between development phases are becoming an artifact of outdated tools and methods. The information age allows us to treat drug development as a continuous process—for example, identifying best doses with a high degree of confidence and then proceeding directly into confirmatory studies. A more continuous development process would also be more responsive than conventional methods to a scientific imperative: to take prompt advantage of new information and techniques to push the frontiers of knowledge. Routine acceptance of intentional delays in the acquisition of knowledge seems at odds with this imperative.

Pauses last from several months for phase I-II transitions to more than a year for phase II-III changeovers. These long between-phase pauses have serious repercussions. Delays make patients wait for improved treatments, tie up development funds, and transform potential market leaders into marginal late entrants in a product category. Pauses may even allow windows of opportunity to slam shut. Throughout any pauses, long or short, the patent clock ticks down and value dissipates.

The tasks performed in conventional between-phase pauses are as important as ever. These tasks include holding discussions with regulators that focus on the interpretation of findings and the design of subsequent studies. Pauses can also allow exploration of unanticipated findings, pursuit of additional funding, producing and packaging necessary drug supplies, and identifying investigational sites. The need to reach agreement with regulators on essential aspects of confirmatory studies before proceeding remains absolute.

When to Consider Seamless Studies

While the tasks performed during between-phase pauses remain important, the argument for always performing all such tasks during long hiatus periods is less convincing. Some development programs seem particularly amenable to combined-phase studies. The programs that can best combine phases usually involve product classes for which the path to market is relatively well defined. In most cases, other drugs in the same therapeutic class have previously won approval. Regulatory agencies generally publish guidance documents for common classes of drugs that outline the development requirements for the class. Relatively short-term outcomes for both safety and efficacy also increase the feasibility of combining phases. Finally, there may be relevant data from other drugs and experience from other trials in the same class that can provide guidance for designing a combined study that achieves all the objectives formerly divided between two separate trials with a pause between. On the other hand, when testing new chemical entities (NCEs) and new indications for existing drugs, combining phases may be more problematic. When both the therapeutic agent and the trial design are novel, researchers and regulators alike may be less certain of how to meet all the informational goals in a single study.

One area that seems particularly well suited to combined-phase studies and rapid transitions is oncology. The search for improved treatments is often urgent. With many therapeutic agents in oncology, it is unethical to perform early toxicity testing on healthy subjects. In many cases, the most sensible and humane approach when testing for toxicity on diseased patients is to gather data on efficacy as well and to hope that the test drug will improve the outlook for patients in the study. Another factor conducive to combined-phase studies in oncology is the availability of well-defined surrogate markers such as tumor response.

Regardless of the therapeutic category, seamless transitions require careful planning. There is an absolute requirement for consideration from the outset of all elements and steps required for each phase involved in the combination. This includes logistical issues as well as informational requirements.

It is worth noting that there is a fallback position from a seamless design—reverting to a more conventional process. As with any clinical program, plans may not always foresee and address all possible outcomes. If surprising twists and turns demand a period of analysis and reflection, a seamless design can impose a delay before implementing the next study. For example, consider a planned phase I/II seamless design that has completed safety testing and quickly initiated several cohorts with different dosing arms. If follow-up to the first phase suggests one or more patients treated during the toxicity finding may be experiencing a delayed but significant side effect from the previous trial, study managers could delay the initiation of phase II activities. This would allow devoting more time to studying the patients treated in phase I and consideration of appropriate next steps. The penalty for abandoning the seamless design would be negligible because, if testing of the drug continued in phase II after a pause, the efficiency would be the same as that of planning and conducting two separate trials. Adaptive designs allow responding more nimbly to circumstances encountered during trials. In this instance, the correct nimble response would be reconsidering the seamless design based on the unforeseen information on toxicity from the previous study. This is in the adaptive spirit even if it means abandoning a seamless design.

Seamless Phase I/Phase II Trials

Although the scale of studies combining phases I and II is relatively small, a combined study still involves greater complexity than two separate studies. At the least, such combination trials require more preparation for contingencies. Since phase I generally focuses on safety and collects little or no efficacy data, the transition to a dose-finding effort that emphasizes efficacy includes different measures, a different observation period, and differences in other key design elements. This shift in focus divides the single trial into two stages, but the trial remains seamless in the sense that it does not require a pause to analyze data and initiate planning of a new study de novo. Nevertheless, there is a transition, and trial managers must be prepared to manage it.

Key factors demanding careful planning and management in seamless studies include:

- drug supply: ensuring that the right amount is available in the right dosing and packaging requires comparing manufacturing and packaging lead times and possibly considerations such as assessing the merits of drugs in bottles versus blister packaging;
- site preparation: identifying sites for the larger study, IRB and other submissions, CRF preparations;
- timeliness of data availability and analysis;
- internal decision making in dose selection.

Case Study 4-5 describes a seamless phase I/phase II study of a treatment combining two chemotherapeutic agents for pancreatic cancer. The design includes provision for both early stopping and selecting a dose to continue into phase II.

Case Study 4-5: Phase I/II study of gemcitabine in combination chemotherapy with raltitrexed in pancreatic adenocarcinoma

Phase I dose escalation combined with phase II evaluation of efficacy and safety[10]

This combination phase I/phase II study sought both to define MTD and to find evidence of clinical benefit. Previous studies indicated gemcitabine had good tolerability and raltitrexed had manageable toxicity. The dose-escalation portion of the study treated patients in a 3+3 design, escalating dose if no patients experienced DLT within 21 days from start of treatment. Patients who did not recover sufficiently from toxicity within 21 days were withdrawn from the study. If one or more patients in a cohort experienced DLT, the study added three more patients at the same dose. If 2 patients then experienced DLT, that established the dosing level as the MTD and the next lower level as the therapeutic dose. Because of severity of side effects, the study reduced the doses of patients who met criteria for recovery to 75% of MTD for the remaining treatment cycles.

Criteria for moving to phase II were treating at least 30 patients in phase I and having more than 4 patients show clinical benefit. If 4 or fewer patients responded to treatment, the study would stop for futility. Otherwise, the study would transition to phase II. For the phase II portion of the trial, sample size was determined using the Simon two-stage minimax design allowing for early termination if the treatment failed to provide sufficient benefit.[3] The sample size for phase II was set at 41; the study was to enroll additional patients until it reached that number.

The study met the criteria for moving to phase II testing, with 6 patients showing clinical benefit. The study successfully made the transition from phase I to phase II testing and continued as planned. However, patients experienced 15 serious adverse events. The investigators decided to stop the study without completing phase II.

Although this study failed to complete phase II, it did accelerate development by allowing a rapid transition between phases. Thus, the study represents an instance of an adaptive design allowing earlier identification of a drug candidate as unsuccessful. The drug candidate "failed faster" than would have been the case with a gap between phase I and phase II testing.

Seamless Phase II/Phase III Trials

The stakes in the later stages of the development process are high. The scale is greater and delays can have profound consequences, such as allowing competitive products to reach the market first. In view of the high stakes, managers should consider whether pausing between studies is a matter of routine or a reasoned choice. Treating phase II and follow-on phase III studies as separate endeavors has disadvantages. For example, it requires initiating two startup processes, building two recruiting operations, and enrolling two separate study populations that may differ in unforeseen ways.

The main benefit of seamlessly combining phases II and III is saving time. The combined approach allows going through the startup process just once. It provides a head start on recruiting investigators and patients for confirmatory testing. Combined studies have a single protocol covering the two phases, a single CRF, and a single process for the drug's development, review, and approval.

Similarities in the design and execution of phase II and phase III studies simplify making a "seamless" transition between the two phases. While studies in these two phases differ chiefly in the number of dosing arms and the time required for observation, most of the evaluations, procedures, and assessments are or can be the same. With careful planning, it may be possible to use data on arms carried over from phase II in the final analysis of confirmatory testing.

However, there are times when important differences between phases would complicate seamless combinations. Some confirmatory studies involve different or more extensive evaluations, such as extended observation for safety or infrequent events. For example, cardiac conduction or ocular issues may require testing greater numbers of patients or observing patients for longer periods. Events in specific subpopulations may require particular attention. If there are such differences between phases, study planners must consider the implications before committing to seamless designs. Nevertheless, the similarity between phase II and phase III studies is often great enough to allow a truly seamless transition, with no stop before initiating phase III.

Pruning Treatment Arms

A combined phase II and phase III study must first establish a number of dosing arms and then prune those to the most suitable doses for the confirmatory phase based on the data available at an interim look. The approach used for interim analysis may allow selecting hypotheses for the confirmatory stage.[11] Another option for combining phase II and phase III trials is use of adaptive randomization to increase allocation of patients to the most promising treatment arms—those most likely to continue into phase III.[12]

Because key elements such as CRFs, databases, and EDC systems are already in place, the transition to confirmatory testing consists primarily of expansion rather than creation de novo. If trial data justifies continuation into the confirmatory portion, the degree of confidence about the best doses to carry forward determines the timing of the transition. At that point, the study brings additional sites online and greatly expands recruiting efforts. In addition, depending on the urgency and an assessment of the strength of the data at an interim look, the sponsor may decide to initiate a second confirmatory study simultaneously.

Figure 4-3 contrasts a seamless adaptive phase II/III trial with the conventional approach of conducting two separate trials.

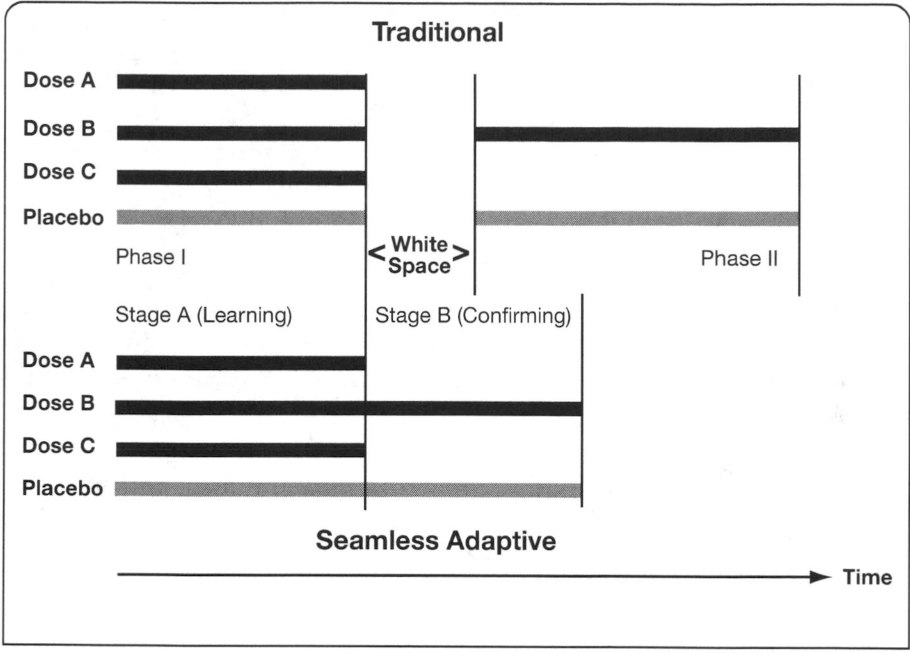

Figure 4-3. A seamless phase II/III trial moves directly from a process identifying the best dose or doses to a confirmatory trial using the selected doses.
Source: Thomas 2007.[4]

Planning Issues in Seamless Trials

Planning and executing an undertaking as complex as a seamless phase II–phase III trial presents significant challenges. Advanced analysis must address the issues that would ordinarily receive separate attention in planning two studies. One challenge is securing regulatory agreement from the outset, with sponsors and regulators resolving key issues before study initiation. Key considerations include design elements, such as sample-size reestimation, as well as how to effect the transition between the two phases.

Initial planning must take particular care to specify what to do in each contingency. Simulations allow study planners to model possible outcomes and analyze the ramifications based on a variety of assumptions. Plans must also address complex statistical issues such as those involved in the possible combination of some data from the dose-finding and confirmatory portions of the combined trial. Study planning must ensure that the protocol and CRF address the objectives of both stages of the combined study.

Scaling up logistics for the transition to phase III is another issue requiring close attention in study planning.

Study planners must determine two samples sizes for a seamless trial, one to meet the needs of each stage. Since the second stage depends on the results of the first, simulation can help with preliminary exploration of sample size, statistical power, and requirements for controlling type 1 error. Information collected during the dose-selection stage can serve as the basis for refining sample-size calculations. The major procedural change in the combined trial usually concerns enrolling additional patients. Patients from the dose-finding stage who received the doses selected for the confirmatory stage usually continue to take the same dose rather than undergoing a second randomization. The study may continue providing follow-up on patients from terminated dose-finding arms.

The final analysis of doses carried forward into the confirmatory stage can include patients from both stages. Combining data from the two stages of the trial requires a technique such as combination tests to control the type 1 error rate for the comparison of the test drug with the control, regardless of the method used to select the doses for the confirmatory stage. One of the most common approaches to controlling error is to combine *p*-values from the two stages. The final statistical analysis for the combined data from the learning and confirmatory phases is likely to be complex (ref. 13, p. 171). Exclusion of bias demands careful attention to a variety of issues, including multiplicity from the selection process and limiting the information revealed by or inferred from an interim analysis. Combining phases raises many other issues, such as providing for an IRB and ensuring timely availability of appropriate consent forms and study materials. Bringing all the necessary components together is no small task.

Although rolling a phase II study into phase III requires great effort, the benefit is likely to be considerably greater. Seamless phase II/phase III studies may reduce development time by a year or more and reduce costs by millions of dollars. With careful planning and management, the risks of combining phases II and III are low.

Case Study 4-6 describes the ASTIN seamless phase II/phase III trial of a new stroke treatment. The design starts with Bayesian dose finding, but the same statistical framework also allows combining phases II and III. Proceeding to phase III depends on developing satisfactory evidence of dose response rather than waiting for the end of a fixed period devoted to phase II.

Case Study 4-6: The ASTIN trial of a neutrophil inhibitory factor as a treatment for acute stroke

Seamless combined phase II dose finding and phase III confirmatory trial using Bayesian methods[14–16]

The Acute Stroke Therapy by Inhibition of Neutrophils (ASTIN) trial was an adaptive phase II dose-response study seeking to establish whether the test agent improves prospects of recovery from acute ischemic stroke. Following identification of doses, the ASTIN trial design provided for continuing to the confirmatory stage within the framework of a single trial. As soon as data established response to the drug and provided sufficient understanding of dose response, the trial would switch to a confirmatory phase with balanced randomization between the identified effective dose and placebo. There would be no delay between phases and no delay in enrolling patients.

Because regulatory review of confirmatory trials relies on analysis of frequentist statistics, the trial used techniques to predict statistical significance in frequentist terms. Study planners set sample size to ensure statistically significant findings using frequentist techniques.

Adaptive methods allowed the study to explore a wider range of doses at finer intervals and thus to acquire superior knowledge about the properties of the test drug. The combination of real-time capture of efficacy data and the Bayesian statistical methods allowed continuous reassessment of the dose response. Continuously updated dose-response information provided the basis for randomizing patients to one of 15 possible doses or placebo using a double-blind procedure.

The design also provided for early termination for either efficacy or futility. The study defined the primary endpoint as change from baseline on the Scandinavian Stroke Scale (SSS) measured up to day 90. The study enrolled 966 acute stroke patients treated within six hours of the onset of stroke symptoms. The trial stopped early based on a 0.89 Bayesian posterior probability of futility.

The performance of the test drug in this seamless study proved disappointing. However, the adaptive design allowed early termination, which saved an estimated $2 million.

A recently initiated combined phase II/phase III study of a recombinant fusion protein as a treatment of systemic lupus erythematosus seeks to identify the better of two test doses for continuation into a confirmatory trial and regulatory submission. (See Case Study 4-7.) The goal is to suppress response on an index of lupus activity and then to measure success in terms of the proportion of patients who avoid flare-ups as measured by the same index.

Case Study 4-7: Combined phase II/III confirmatory study in generalized systemic lupus erythematosus

Phase II dose selection followed by phase III confirmatory trial[17]

This double-blind randomized efficacy study with parallel assignment will collect final data on the primary outcome measure in January 2011 or later. The plan calls for a phase II portion of the trial testing 75 mg and 150 mg subcutaneous doses of atacicept, a recombinant fusion protein, against placebo. The planned sample size is approximately 510.

Patients in each of the three arms will receive their respective doses or placebo twice a week for 4 weeks and then continue treatment weekly for 48 weeks. Key inclusion criteria include BILAG (British Isles Lupus Assessment Group) flare A or B (designations in a lupus activity response index) at screening requiring change in corticosteroids. If treatment reduces patient scores to C or D on the index, the primary outcome measure will be the proportion of patients who experience a new flare A or B during the 52-week period of treatment. The study will assess patients monthly. Assessment will continue until 24 weeks after last dose. If one of the doses demonstrates sufficient efficacy as measured by BILAG, that dose will continue into a phase III confirmatory trial.

The initiation of this study illustrates the trend toward accelerating drug development by proceeding directly from dose finding into confirmatory testing.

Seamless phase II/III trials can provide important advantages beyond condensing timelines and reducing costs. The information from a seamless phase II/III study can accelerate a program by allowing earlier initiation of a second confirmatory phase III trial and earlier acquisition of long-term safety data to support a regulatory filing. Figure 4-4 shows a sequence of trials providing these benefits.

Phase I-II-III Designs

The ability to continue a phase I trial directly into phase II and a phase II trial directly into phase III suggests the possibility of combining all three phases into one seamless study. Such a combined study would treat clinical development as a continuous process of acquiring all the information

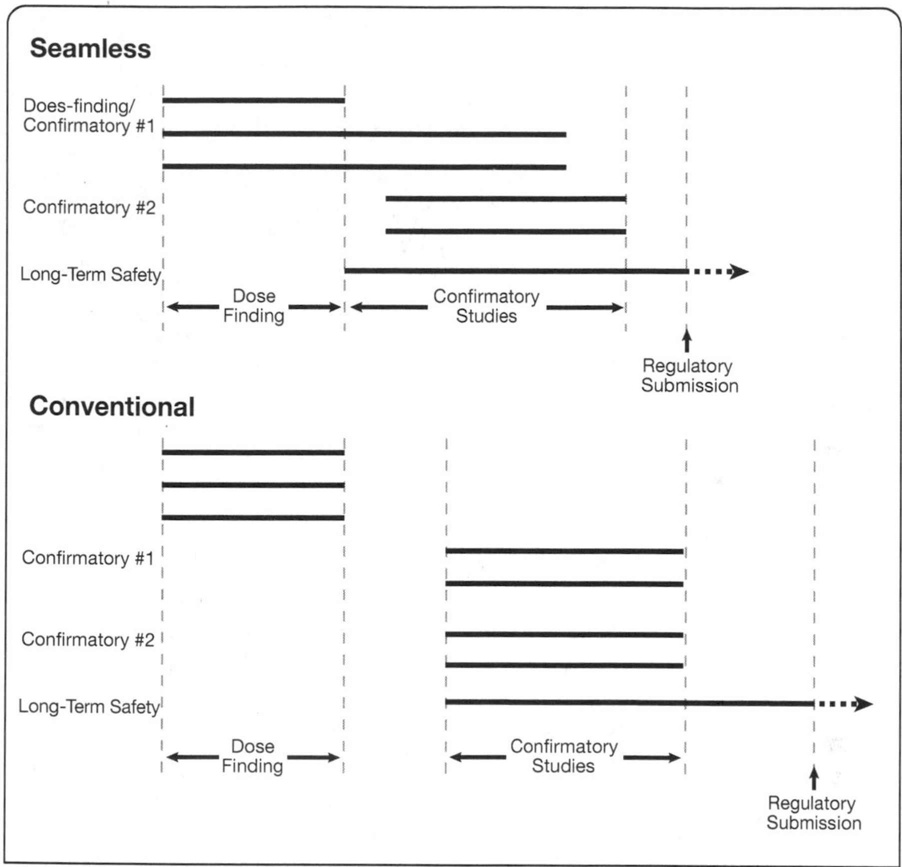

Figure 4-4. A seamless phase II/III trial is is more efficient than a traditional approach with two distinct trials, allows a second confirmatory (phase III) study to be started earlier, and provides earlier long-term safety information. An important difference is adaptive's ability to minimize or eliminate between-study pauses, which can be substantial.

necessary for a regulatory submission. The design of the ASTIN study incorporates elements of all three conventional phases, from safety to the confirmatory phase. The ASTIN trial assessed safety and identified doses for confirmatory testing. The trial did not continue into the confirmatory phase because the test drug did not work.

However, one development program has already successfully combined all three phases in a single trial. If combining two phases increases the complexity of planning, adding a third phase presents planners with even greater challenges. Case Study 4-8 illustrates.

Case Study 4-8: Seamless phase I-II-III design for unidentified GI indication

Multiple adaptive techniques with CRM dose finding and subsequent dose pruning with multiple interim analyses (Health Decisions, Inc.)

For a GI indication, this study involved relatively short-term efficacy and safety issues. A conventional single ascending dose study initiated the portion of the trial focused on determining toxicity. The seamless portion began with a second phase I study, examining both toxicity and short-term efficacy. This design included a variable number of subjects per arm. The second study used a CRM approach to select a starting dose at which available dose-response information suggested a 40% probability of toxicity. Since the product is an antibody, there was an expectation that defining toxicity would be difficult. Therefore, the primary indicator was one of immunologic function.

The dose-finding portion of the study adjusted the dose up or down depending on toxicity until response data defined an approximate dose-response curve. At each iteration, the study doubled the number of subjects in the groups treated. However, the study held the number of subjects for the comparator group constant after reaching a predetermined size. This portion of the study enrolled patients with poorly controlled cases of the GI indication. The study performed safety assessments for the first two weeks and continued another two weeks to assess efficacy. By the end of this portion, the study had reasonably defined both safety and toxicity. It had also identified six arms for progression to dose finding.

The dose-finding portion used arms of fixed size and included multiple interim analyses. Although there was formal statistical testing at several points, the protocol allowed terminating arms based on collective judgment of the sponsor's team. The target for phase III was to retain two active treatment arms and one standard-treatment comparator. Within several months, study managers decided to drop two active treatment arms, primarily on efficacy grounds. The study rapidly expanded the remaining arms and added a second confirmatory study using additional sites. The plan going forward included a sample-size reestimation when the study had accumulated half the data anticipated for phase III.

This study illustrates progress toward treating development as a continuum, with the speed of development limited less by the conventional division of testing than by the ability to acquire the knowledge necessary to proceed to the next step.

Adaptive Randomization

What can change: ratio for allocation of patients to treatment arms

Criteria for change: evidence of superior arm, imbalance of covariates among arms, chance deviation from intended allocation ratio

Adaptive randomization alters the probability of patient allocation to different arms in order to meet a variety of objectives. For example, if accumulating trial data shows one arm to be more desirable and more likely to continue into additional testing, the randomization procedure may increase the probability of allocating patients to that arm. At the outset, all treatment arms have the same allocation ratio. As information on outcomes increases, the randomization ratio can change to achieve a variety of objectives, including:

- increasing the likelihood of assignment to the more effective or safe treatment (response-adaptive randomization);
- balancing covariates (risk factors that modify the probability of an outcome) across different treatment arms (covariate-adaptive randomization);
- correcting a chance deviation from the intended allocation ratio (treatment-adaptive randomization)(ref. 13, p.171).

Some adaptive randomization procedures combine multiple methods. Covariate-adjusted response-adaptive randomization considers the responses of previous patients to treatment, previous patient covariates, and the covariates of the patient awaiting randomization (ref. 18, pp. 4, 6, 7).

Adaptive randomization obviously presents greater complexity than maintaining fixed, equal allocation to each treatment arm for the life of the study, regardless of whether study data shows some arms to be less effective or less safe. However, the advantages justify the effort. For example, adaptive randomization has clear ethical advantages over maintaining fixed allocation ratios despite evidence of lesser efficacy or safety. Furthermore, when data shows an imbalance in covariates between treatment groups, continuing with a fixed allocation procedure may reduce the ability to draw valid inferences about differences in treatment effect. Similarly, continuing with a fixed allocation approach despite the development of imbalances in the actual size of treatment groups could undermine statistical power and thus jeopardize the validity of a trial.

Response-Adaptive Randomization

Response-adaptive randomization typically changes the proportion of patients allocated to an arm based on the likelihood of favorable outcome for the treatment given that arm. As accumulating data shows a more favorable outcome for one arm, allocation of patients to that arm increases. The benefit for patients is obvious—more of them get the treatment that appears likely to prove best.

There is a variety of different algorithms for response-adaptive randomization (ref. 13, pp. 58–60).The most common is the randomized play-the-winner scheme. This requires knowing the outcome for the previous patient before randomizing the next patient to a treatment group. If the treatment for the preceding patient has a positive outcome, an additional "ball" representing that patient's treatment group goes into the randomization pool or "urn." If the outcome of treatment for the preceding patient is negative, the number of balls representing the treatment group remains as before. At the outset, the figurative urn contains equal numbers of balls of each color, with each color representing a different treatment group. Over time, the urn contains more and more balls with colors representing the arms with the more beneficial treatment, resulting in allocation of more patients to the most promising treatments.

Response-adaptive randomization allows the collection of more data on patient response to the test drug at the dose levels that the sponsor is likely to submit for regulatory approval. This offers the possibility of acquiring greater knowledge about the drug's properties in the doses that prescribing information for physicians is most likely to recommend. The superior prescribing information benefits both physicians and patients. More and better information on these doses may also aid the deliberations of regulators.

Other Forms of Adaptive Randomization

As the name suggests, covariate-adaptive randomization seeks to balance covariates across treatment groups. Weighting of the randomization procedure increases allocation of patients with certain covariates to treatment groups in which these covariates are underrepresented (ref. 13, pp. 55–59; ref. 18, p. 6). (In practice, mathematical techniques such as multivariable analysis can also address imbalances in covariates.)

Treatment-adaptive randomization uses a variety of weighting schemes to balance the number of patients assigned to each treatment group in order to correct for lagging membership. One approach is to use an algorithm that imitates the behavior of a coin designed to favor the treatment group in question (ref. 13, pp. 53–55).

One Bayesian technique for adaptive randomization allocates patients to a specific arm in proportion to the continuously calculated degree of promise it shows relative to other arms—the posterior probability of the dose for that arm proving best at the end of the trial. As results for each treatment accumulate, the allocation ratio increasingly favors the most promising treatment. A predetermined state defines study completion. For example, if a study begins with a 1:1 randomization scheme but then adds a ball to the randomization urn for each successful outcome, the urn increasingly favors the successful arm. With a Bayesian approach, planners might deem a study complete when randomization assigns 95% or some other specific proportion of patients to a particular arm, reflecting the preponderance of successful treatments experienced by patients previously assigned to that arm.

Adaptive randomization requires special infrastructure: a centralized randomization system that can allocate an enrolling patient in real time based on the latest information. This is in addition to basic requirements for all adaptive techniques, such as efficient data capture and cleaning. A centralized, real-time randomization mechanism also increases efficiency. It provides an ideal way to cut off enrollment promptly after reaching the target population size. This eliminates unnecessary effort, expense, and patient exposure associated with systems that are incapable of assessing and controlling enrollment in real time. (Case Study 4-3 provides an example of a study that enrolled more than 200 patients in excess of what sample-size reestimation showed to be necessary.)

The trial described in Case Study 4-9 used one of the most well established approaches to adaptive randomization, the Pocock-Simon biased-coin randomization procedure.[19]

Case Study 4-9: The VANQWISH (Veterans Affairs Non-Q-Wave Infarction Strategies In-Hospital) trial

Adaptive randomization for balance by treatment center and stratifying variables[20]

This study of non-Q-wave myocardial infarction patients following thrombolytic therapy compared outcomes of patients randomized to receive either invasive or conservative postinfarct assessment strategies. Adaptive randomization increased the probability of balance between the two tested strategies by treatment center and by five stratifying variables. Randomization took place 24–48 hours after the onset of infarction.

The study controlled for between-center differences and minimized imbalances among treatment groups within levels of each prognostic factor. After determining the degree of imbalance for each prognostic factor, the Pocock-Simon algorithm hypothetically assigns each successive subject to each treatment arm, assesses the resulting balance among arms, and then assigns the subject to whichever treatment arm minimizes imbalances. This approach statistically balances risk factors to allow an unbiased estimate of the effect of the two postinfarct assessment strategies.

Another well-established adaptive randomization approach is the urn-adaptive biased-coin method of Wei and Lachin.[21] This method achieves balance among treatment groups in smaller populations, while in studies with larger populations it has the highly desirable property of approaching complete randomization. Case Study 4-10 describes a confirmatory trial of a novel T-cell modulator as a treatment for plaque psoriasis.

Case Study 4-10: Phase III trial of efalizumab as a treatment for plaque psoriasis

Adaptive randomization with the urn-adaptive biased-coin method to achieve balance by treatment center and stratifying variables

This phase III trial assessed efalizumab (Genentech's Raptiva), a novel T-cell modulator, as a treatment for plaque psoriasis. The urn-adaptive biased-coin method ensured balance within several subgroups defined according to the baseline psoriasis area-and-severity index, previous systemic treatment for psoriasis, and investigational site.

The double-blind, multicenter, randomized study with placebo control randomized 597 patients tc treatment with efalizumab or placebo for a period of 12 weeks. Based on response at that time, patients received an additional 12 weeks of treatment with efalizumab or placebo. The study stopped treatments at week 24. Thereafter, the study followed subjects for an additional 12 weeks. The first treatment phase assigned patients in ratios of 2:2:1 to a low dose of the test therapeutic agent, a higher dose, or placebo.

Response-adaptive randomization in a leukemia study progressively shifted the randomization of patients to the most favorable treatment arm (Case Study 4-11).

Case Study 4-11: Study of three combination chemotherapeutic regimens in older untreated patients with adverse karyotype acute myeloid leukemia

Response-adaptive randomization with Bayesian allocation rule[22]

This study started with equal randomization to three arms but progressively allocated more patients to the more effective treatments. The study defined success as complete remission within 49 days of starting treatment.

The study labeled the three treatment arms IA, TA, and TI. Thirty-four patients received treatment. The randomization procedure recalculated probabilities for the arms with the entry of each new patient. The percentage of patients allocated to arm TA increased to 59% by the time of the enrollment of patient 24, with the probability of assignment to TI reduced to 7% and the probability of assignment to IA remaining at 33⅓%. However, success rates had changed when patient 25 enrolled. They were 55% with IA, 43% with TA, and 0% with TI. At that point, allocation stopped for treatment arm TI and shifted heavily in favor of arm IA. However, the responses of three patients were unknown at that time. Probability of randomization to IA reached 96% with the enrollment of the 34th patient. Thus, the randomization procedure allocated more patients to the active control late in the trial.

Remission rates after 49 days were 55% for the IA arm, 27% for the TA arm, and 0% for the TI arm. However, follow-up beyond the 49-day period found that three complete remissions occurred after the period included in the definition of successful response. Based on these additional remissions, the adjusted final remission rates were 55%, 45%, and 20%, respectively, for the three arms. The study established a 70% probability that TA was inferior to IA, with a probability of 5% that TA would have a remission rate 20% higher than IA.

The decision rules reflected a relatively high probability of falsely declaring test arms superior to the active control. This allowed a greater probability of correctly selecting the test arms if they were truly superior. Despite this, the study concluded that neither of the other arms was superior to arm IA, a combination of idarubicin and cytarabine (ara-C).

Other Types of Design Adaptations

Today's adaptive trials predominantly employ sample-size reestimation and dose-finding techniques. These techniques are here to stay. However, the adaptive toolbox is growing. Research continues to hone existing adaptive techniques and identify new techniques to allow acquisition of greater knowledge and to achieve greater efficiency.

One potentially important class of adaptive techniques allows extending the period of assessment and decision making in a trial. For example, such an adaptation may allow changing the test hypothesis from superiority to noninferiority. In principle, trial data could support a regulatory filing for approval based on noninferiority while the trial continues to collect data in the hope of later demonstrating superiority. Other adaptations allow redesigning multiple endpoints to update correlations or change the hierarchical order. It is also possible to establish a decision rule with criteria for determining whether to refocus the study on a predetermined subpopulation.

Noninferiority-to-Superiority Design

There is often interplay between the imperative to get a product to market as quickly as possible and the importance of establishing the superiority of that new product to existing options. Demonstrating superiority offers the greatest potential in the marketplace, and products often begin development with the promise of superiority to existing choices. However, sometimes evidence for equivalence—noninferiority in statistical terms—becomes clear while superiority remains in doubt, even in late-stage testing. The sponsor may decide to bring the product to market based on noninferiority, perhaps in a subpopulation or with the benefit of causing fewer adverse effects.

Other factors being equal, studies for establishing noninferiority have the advantage of requiring smaller sample sizes. This increases the appeal of beginning the approval process immediately after crossing the noninferiority threshold but continuing or expanding the study to establish superiority. Generally, a midcourse check, such as that performed with a sample-size reestimation, will provide a good sense of whether a new product is superior to its comparator and, if so, by how much. Based on this information, the easiest and most straightforward course midstudy or midprogram is to declare the goal of noninferiority or superiority.

Running a study that evaluates both noninferiority and superiority requires detailed regulatory discussions. Careful control of type 1 error is essential. Programs that elect to meet the immediate goal of noninferiority and continue to demonstrate superiority require negotiations with regulatory authorities to set individual parameters such as the margin of noninferiority. This is typically 10%, but in some cases, a product wins approval despite efficacy that is inferior by as much as 30%. For example, antibiotics typically have more permissive noninferiority requirements than oncology products.

Adaptive Hypotheses and Subpopulations

Focus on subpopulations in clinical research is increasing, especially with genetic and other markers predicting strength of outcomes. Subpopulation analysis can yield striking information. Early clinical trials of sepsis drugs failed uniformly in the population as a whole, but analysis of subpopulations often revealed success in certain groups. Similarly, early development showed that herceptin worked well only in breast cancer patients who carry the *HER2* gene. Without question, markers will play an important role in identifying subpopulations in future research. Researchers and clinical practitioners will take advantage of not only genetic markers but also metabolic and other types of markers. The use of multiple markers offers still greater potential in a manner resembling the ability of multivariable analyses to consider many potential predictors simultaneously. In later development, regulatory authorities have sometimes allowed dropping subpopulations. Narrowing the indication can increase the chances of program success.

Studies, especially early studies, sometimes produce data that study planners did not anticipate, perhaps raising entirely unanticipated hypotheses. The peripheral vasodilator minoxidil started development as an antihypertensive agent. The serendipitous observation that topical application of minoxidil promotes hair growth had no apparent connection with the initial interests of the investigators. Resetting the target indication and population ultimately made minoxidil the first drug approved by the FDA for male-pattern hair loss. (The drug did also win approval as an oral antihypertensive.)

The idea of focusing development efforts on groups where the therapeutic effect is strongest has great appeal, both ethical and strategic. The conventional approach to identification of subpopulations is to conduct an exploratory study, to confirm its findings in a phase II study, then to confirm phase II findings in a phase III study. An adaptive approach enables initiation of an exploratory study as a seamless phase II/III study, conducting midcourse subpopulation analysis, then dropping less effective groups and continuing or expanding the study.[23] This staged approach can first allow a decision about which, if any, subpopulations to keep and which to drop, as demonstrated in Case Study 4-12. The second stage has the objective of demonstrating superiority.

Case Study 4-12: Advanced/metastatic oncology product

Adaptive selection of hypothesis, narrowing focus of development program[24]

Evaluation of a new oncology drug defined superior efficacy as at least 23% greater progression-free survival than the control arm. The study set the target number of events at 918 in the full population or 640 in a subpopulation of interest. Maximum total sample size was 1,200 patients.

The first interim analysis reviewed efficacy and futility utilizing 170 events (~19% of target full-population events). Timing of the review allowed accumulating enough information for decision making as well as recruiting enough patients in stage 2. The second interim analysis considered efficacy alone. This classical interim analysis was added to the initial two-stage adaptive design and was scheduled to take place after accumulation of 551 full-population events, or, if a subpopulation was selected, 384 events in the subpopulation (60% of target number of events, halfway through stage 2).

A series of power simulations explored different scenarios and determined the power for each. The first scenario was that all patients benefit equally from treatment; the second that only a subpopulation with a specific biomarker benefits. Within the second scenario, the simulations explored a range of values for the proportion of the total population represented by the subpopulation. The design of the final study would depend on results of the interim analysis: if that reflected a substantially greater effect in the subpopulation, then the study would either be restricted to that subpopulation or require inclusion of a certain proportion of patients from that subpopulation. If interim results did not show substantially greater effect in the subpopulation, the study would recruit more broadly.

The approach allowed combining data on stage 1 patients with data on stage 2 patients for final analysis. Thus, the stage 1 patients contributed to both phase II and III objectives. The study design provided an equal or greater probability of success than a conventional phase III design that would have either ignored the subpopulation or tested the hypothesis of a difference on the full population.

The program identified the subpopulation in a concurrent but separate exploratory trial. This approach allowed phase III to start approximately one to two years earlier. It also required approximately 200 fewer patients than the conventional approach.

Treatment Switching

The treatment of some diseases changes based on initial outcomes. For example, oncology studies involve initial treatment with one drug or regimen and, based on disease progression, change to another. Treatment switching depends on initial response. Survival analysis must therefore consider both the initial and postprogression marker for survival. Analysis may become still more complex if there is a third progression that affects the choice of treatment provided. In simple terms, treatment-switching studies "start" with the first switch, and the outcome is either disease progression or death. Each assessment involving a decision about treatment requires mapping out the possibilities. Such complex studies are rare because of both statistical and operational challenges.

Conclusions

The ability to use study data to make midcourse design changes enables much greater efficiency than the conventional wait-and-see approach to clinical research. The case studies in this chapter show that techniques for adapting study designs in midcourse have already increased speed, efficiency or both in a variety of studies. While fast moving adaptive programs demand more detailed planning and more active decision making, there is little downside to the employment of these adaptive techniques. In the worst case, efficiency matches that of conventional studies.

Importantly, the benefits of design adaptations extend beyond economics. They touch real people. Adaptive techniques can reduce the number of patients exposed to less effective or less safe doses during the course of development. Reducing development time accelerates the delivery of effective new drugs to patients who need them. Reducing development costs can help make new drugs more affordable without compromising industry resources. The next chapter shows how operational adaptations provide equally impressive gains in efficiency, with comparable benefits for the industry and the public.

References

1 Chuang-Stein C, Anderson K, Gallo P, Collins S. Sample size reestimation: a review and recommendations. Drug Inf J. 2006;40:475–84.

2 Lan KKG, DeMets DL. Discrete sequential boundaries for clinical trials. Biometrika. 1983;70:659–63.

3 Simon R. Optimal two-stage designs for phase II clinical trials. Control Clin Trials. 1989;10:1–10.

4 Thomas P. The adaptive design: issues in current research and implementation. Presentation at fourth national congress of the Società Italiana di Statistica Medica ed Epidemiologia Clinica. Feb 2, 2007. Milan, Italy.

5 Anderson K. Adaptive designs: sample size reestimation: a review and recommendations. Presentation to PhRMA Adaptive Designs Workshop. Nov 13, 2006. Bethesda, MD. Available from: http://www.innovation.org/documents/File/Adaptive_Designs_Presentations/13_Anderson_Sample_Size_reestimation_A_review_and_recommendation.pdf.

6 Mehta CR. Design and interim monitoring of flexible clinical trials. Presentation to Eleventh Annual Biopharmaceutical Applied Statistics Symposium. Nov 3–4, 2004. Savannah, GA. Available from: http://www.cytel.com/Papers/bass_11_04.pdf.

7 Taylor AL, et al. Combination of isosorbide dinitrate and hydralazine in blacks with heart failure. NEJM. 2004;351:2049–57.

8 MacDonald TM, et al. Effect on blood pressure of lumiracoxib versus ibuprofen in patients with osteoarthritis and controlled hypertension: a randomized trial. J Hypertension 2008;26:1695–1702.

9 O'Connor CM, et al. Azithromycin for the secondary prevention of coronary heart disease events: the WIZARD study: a randomized controlled trial. JAMA. 2003;290:1459–66.

10 Agnieszka M, et al. Phase I/II study to investigate the use of gemcitabine in combination with raltitrexed in locally advanced or metastatic pancreatic adenocarcinoma. Internet J Oncol [Internet]. 2006 [cited Aug 12, 2008];3(2). Available from: http://www.ispub.com/ostia/index.php?xmlFilePath=journals/ijo/vol3n2/gemcitabine.xml.

11 Bretz F, Schmidli H, König F, Racine A, Maurer W. Confirmatory seamless phase II/III clinical trials with hypotheses selection at interim: general concepts. Biom J. 2006;48:623–34.

12 Wang L, Cui L. Seamless Phase II/III combination study through response adaptive randomization. J Biopharm Stat. 2007;17:1177–87.

13 Chow Shein-Chung, Chang M. Adaptive design methods in clinical trials. Boca Raton, FL: Chapman & Hall/CRC; 2007.

14 Krams M, et al. Acute stroke therapy by inhibition of neutrophils (ASTIN): an adaptive dose-response study of UK-279,276 in acute ischemic stroke. Stroke. 2003;34:2543–8. Available from: http://stroke.ahajournals.org/cgi/content/full/34/11/2543.

15 Berry DA, et al. Adaptive Bayesian designs for dose-ranging drug trials. In: Gatsonis C, et al., editors. Case studies in Bayesian statistics V. New York: Springer-Verlag; 2001. pp. 99–181.

16 Müller P, et al. A Bayesian decision-theoretic dose-finding trial. Decision Anal. 2006;3:197–207.

17 A randomised, double-blind, placebo controlled, multicentre prospective dose-finding phase II/III study with atacicept given subcutaneously to subjects having recently experienced a flare of systemic lupus erythematosus (SLE). In: ClinicalTrials.gov [Internet]. Bethesda (MD): National Library of Medicine (US). Feb 15, 2008. [Cited Aug 12, 2008]. Available from: http://clinicaltrials.gov/ct2/show/NCT00624338.

18 Hu F, Rosenberger W. The theory of response-adaptive randomization in clinical trials. Hoboken, NJ: John Wiley & Sons, 2006.

19 Pocock SJ, Simon R. Sequential treatment assignment with balancing for prognostic factors in the controlled clinical trial. Biometrics. 1975;31:103–15.

20 Wexler L, et al., for the Veterans Affairs Non-Q-Wave Infarction Strategies in Hospital (VANQWISH) Trial Investigators. Non-Q-wave myocardial infarction following thrombolytic therapy: a comparison of outcomes in patients randomized to invasive or conservative post-infarct assessment strategies in the Veterans Affairs Non-Q-Wave Infarction Strategies In-Hospital (VANQWISH) trial. J Am Coll Cardiol. 2001;37:19–25.

21 Wei LJ, Lachin J. Properties of the urn randomization in clinical trials. Control Clin Trials. 1988;9:345–64. [Erratum, Control Clin Trials Mar 1989;10(1):following 126.]

22 Giles F, et al. Adaptive randomized study of idarubicin and cytarabine versus troxacitabine and cytarabine versus troxacitabine and idarubicin in untreated patients 50 years or older with adverse karyotype acute myeloid leukemia. J Clin Oncol. 2003;21:1722–27.

23 Hommel G, Kropf S. Clinical trials with an adaptive choice of hypotheses. Drug Inf J. 2001;35:1423–9.

24 Zuber E, et al. Adaptive seamless designs for subpopulation based on time to event endpoints. Presented at the 5th International Conference on Multiple Comparison Procedures, Vienna, 2007. Available from: http://www.mcp-conference.org/2007/presentations/Zuber_Emmanuel.pdf.

— Chapter 5 —

Operational Adaptations

The capacity for design adaptations depends on the capacity for operational adaptations. Operational adaptations use continuous measurements of the many day-to-day activities that directly and indirectly influence the speed and efficiency of study execution. These measurements allow refinement of operations in many areas, including patient enrollment, data quality, and rapid database and study closure. Operational adaptations thus focus on effective management of studies and programs.

Design and Operational Adaptations

This chapter discusses the individual elements of operational adaptations rather than presenting a comprehensive, integrated effort to optimize an entire study. The examples show a selection from the great variety of ways in which operational adaptations can improve efficiency. Since each study presents unique operational challenges as it unfolds, coping with these challenges requires the ability to think creatively and draw on a wide variety of tools and techniques.

Operational adaptations share many characteristics with design adaptations. Both use current study data to improve efficiency. Both help reduce dead time between studies and phases. Both facilitate a look-ahead capability providing earlier insights for study and program planning. Both also require the same infrastructure.

Common Infrastructure

Design and operational adaptations rely on a common technological infrastructure that rapidly collects, summarizes, and reports information relevant to specific study roles: the right information to the right eyes at the right time. However, infrastructure by itself does not ensure the availability of the timely, accurate information required by the statistical methods used in design adaptations. There must also be the capacity for operational adaptations to ensure that infrastructure and processes actually perform at a high enough level. Figure 5-1 shows how design adaptations rest atop a pyramid of dependencies with technological infrastructure at the base and the capacity for operational adaptations occupying an intermediate layer.

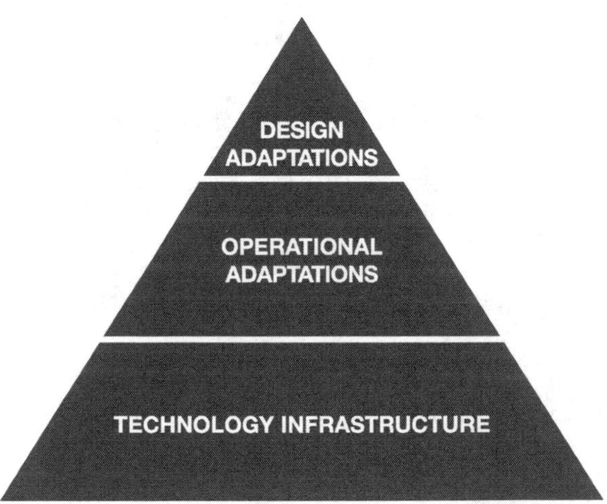

Figure 5-1. Design and operational adaptations rest on the same technological infrastructure. However, design adaptations also depend on operational adaptations that ensure timely availability of clean, accurate data.

Differences between Design and Operational Adaptations

Design adaptations use data collected during a study to refine planning estimates and reduce or eliminate activities that are futile, inferior, or unnecessary. Operational adaptations optimize the execution of a study. A broad range of performance indicators provide a basis for continuous fine-tuning of activities such as patient enrollment, data handling, site monitoring, site closeout, and database lock.

Design and operational adaptations differ not only in focus but also in the number and scope of changes allowed. Design adaptations make infrequent, carefully circumscribed changes. Operational adaptations continuously improve the hundreds or even thousands of activities that determine day-to-day execution of studies and programs, including patient enrollment, site monitoring, site performance, CRF organization and wording, site training, resource allocation, and administration of site payments and study supplies. An area of particular focus is minimizing the rework needed to assure reliable, accurate data.

The Nature and Significance of Operational Adaptations

The main difference between design and operational adaptations is what they change in order to achieve greater efficiency. Operational adaptations also differ from design adaptations in the following ways:

- They are applicable to virtually all studies, though they provide greatest benefits in large, complex studies and programs.
- They involve specific adjustments that are best identified after a study is in progress.
- They leave study design unchanged.
- They do not require regulatory approval.
- They need not be detailed in study protocols, although a protocol may state the intention to identify and implement adaptations in key operations.
- They allow great flexibility as to whether, how, when, and to what extent each operational adaptation is carried out.
- Time and cost savings from operational adaptations, in the aggregate, often exceed those of design adaptations.

The scale of the benefits from operational adaptations bears particular emphasis because the benefit provided by each individual operational adaptation may be small. Nevertheless, the collective effects of numerous operational adaptations can improve the efficiency of a study as much or even more than a successful design adaptation such as sample-size reestimation.

The Current Approach to Operations

Despite the central role of data in clinical research, standard practice still relies on inefficient, error-prone processes to record and manage data. Three related problems characterize the typical approach to handling data in clinical trials:

- Effort focuses on correcting errors, as opposed to identifying and eliminating their causes.
- Standard practice tolerates delays in cleaning, processing, and analyzing data, allowing errors to linger undetected.

- Neither infrastructure nor operating procedures track metrics that reflect the timeliness and quality of work processes.

A recent survey of companies conducting phase III trials found that only half track data errors and patient retention rates. Even fewer track investigator recruitment rates and site retention rates.[1] Only 12% track CRFs collected per monitor-day or patient response to different advertising and marketing approaches for patient recruitment (Figure 5-2)(ref. 1, p. 130). Perhaps most telling, however, is the collective indication that the first step towards improving operations, benchmarking curent practice, is infrequent (Figure 5-3)(ref. 1, p. 132).

Figures 5-2 and 5-3 suggest that clinical studies today make relatively little effort to adapt and optimize study operations.

Implementing Operational Adaptations

By taking full advantage of performance measures, operational adaptations seek to identify as many errors and inefficiencies as possible and eliminate them at the source. The following sections show how operational adaptations improve the efficiency of clinical studies in five general areas:

- enrollment and other site issues;
- data quality issues;
- monitoring;
- study closeout and database lock;
- supporting operations: communications, supplies, and lab results.

Enrollment and Other Site Issues

Although site selection and management probably affect study progress more than any other factor, typical studies devote little systematic attention to these tasks. For example, the essential starting point of good enrollment is good sites, but studies generally choose sites based on casual considerations such as word of mouth, referrals from colleagues, or previous experience. Many studies use site questionnaires, but in a limited manner that focuses on the promised recruitment ability of each site. Experienced managers discount such estimates, often 50% or more. Studies rarely track or assess a variety of performance measures that reflect core capabilities and predict recruitment success.

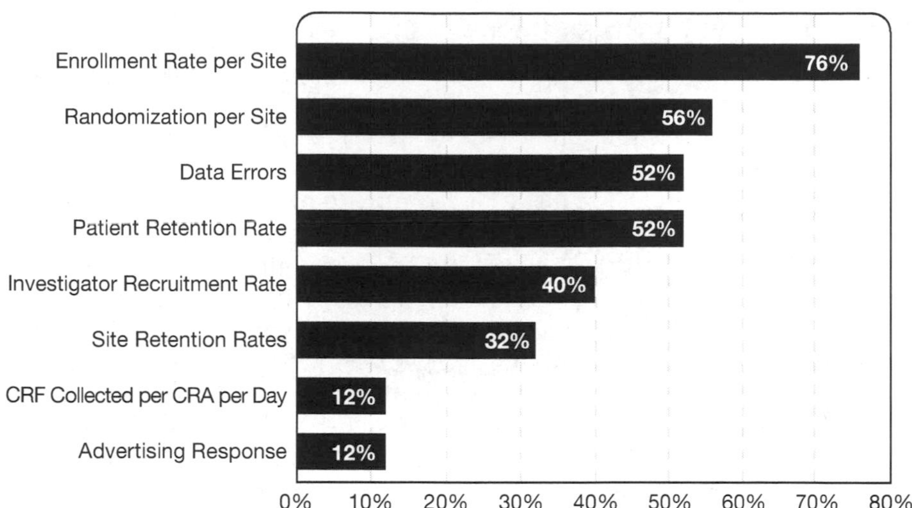

Figure 5-2. Performance measures normally tracked during a phase III clinical trial.

Source: Cutting Edge Information.[1]

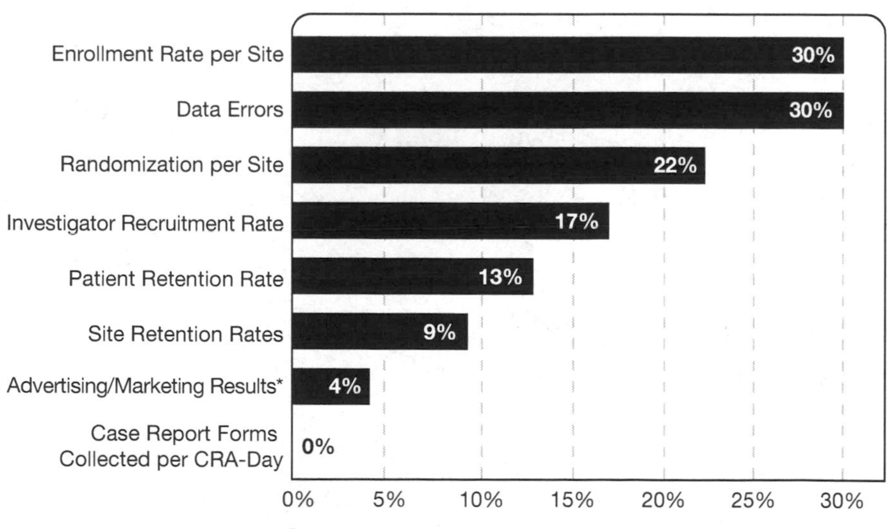

Figure 5-3. Performance measures that bring about changes in operational performance.

Source: Cutting Edge Information.[1]

Aligning Site and Sponsor Interests

Site contracts rarely provide incentives for better performance; many sites see requests for better performance as a demand for extra work without compensation. This situation is common wherever the individuals performing the work receive no financial or other incentives. Academic sites are the leading example. Most studies do little to help sites enroll patients, minimize patients lost to follow-up, submit data on a timely basis, close out sites promptly, and carry out a host of other tasks that can impede study progress. Since measurements tracking performance at such activities are lacking, there is no basis for incentives and disincentives to align the interests of sites with those of the sponsor. Sites receive the same compensation regardless of performance, sometimes despite failing at the most basic task of enrolling patients. Managers cannot compare performance between one site and another, an activity that would allow identifying and encouraging the most and least successful practices. Incentives are a valuable but neglected way to encourage efficiency in critical areas such as submission of data, resolution of queries, and minimization of error rates.

Linking regular payments to timely submission of data and resolution of queries is an excellent way to improve performance. At least one company pays sites according to data received—not only basic CRF data but also data from optional procedures and procedures involving only a subset of patients, such as magnetic resonance imaging (MRI) and lumbar puncture. The company pays sites 80% of the visit payment on receipt of data and the balance upon resolution of queries associated with the data. Another type of incentive provides payment upon completion of the entire set of CRFs for each patient visit. This type of incentive motivates sites to keep up with protocol requirements and focus on patients for whom treatment is lagging or data incomplete. Performance metrics can serve as a basis for such incentives, for disincentives, or for a combination.

Site Selection and Initiation for Adaptive Studies

The ability to manage enrollment adaptively starts with site selection. Site selection should weigh not only the usual qualifications such as how many patients sites say they can enroll, but also the likely ease or difficulty of monitoring study operations at each site. It is helpful to assess how closely the sites monitor their own operations. Does site management take an active or laissez faire approach? Is the managerial style quantitative or seat-of-the-pants? Will the site closely track its efforts to recruit and enroll patients or allow events to run their course? Sites that take a proactive approach to management are likely to have particular aptitude for performing studies that use adaptive techniques. The adaptive approach is all about study management. Sites already disposed to manage in response to changing information will flourish in the adaptive world; if they pay close attention to budgets, timelines, and goals, so much the better.

Online Site Questionnaires

Online questionnaires can collect information that allows study managers to compare sites on uniform criteria. Filling out an online questionnaire is convenient for sites and the study team alike. Online survey tools are readily available, inexpensive, and easy to configure. Spreadsheet analysis of the data collected allows ranking sites and making choices about primary and, if warranted, secondary sites. Open-ended questions allow sites to submit information that might otherwise escape the attention of study managers.

Document Submission

Performance at submitting required documents can serve as a simple but valuable metric to aid in final site selection. The mechanical steps involved in providing study documentation, ranging from 1572s to IRB templates to CRFs to protocols, are straightforward. Efficiency and timeliness in submitting documents at this stage is an important early indicator of likely site performance. Sites that fail to meet document submission deadlines raise a red flag.

Optimizing Enrollment

Available statistics on enrollment performance show overwhelmingly dismal results. According to one report, pharma companies cite patient recruitment as having the greatest impact on the rising cost of clinical development (ref. 1, p. 162). A 2009 Centerwatch survey of sites in four major geographic regions found universal difficulty meeting enrollment targets (Figure 5-4).[2] The percentage of studies enrolling on time was only 10% in the United States, with 68% of studies experiencing delays greater than one month.

The basic requirements for managing enrollment are simple: plan carefully, track progress using timely, relevant indices of performance toward the goal, and refine continuously. These simple requirements often go unmet, as illustrated by a recent statement by a global study manager at a large pharma company:

> *For the most part, when it comes to what's going on in remote sites, I really have no idea—I have to take the word of the local managers about what's done and where the problems lie and how things might be improved. When I do get information, it's often months old.*

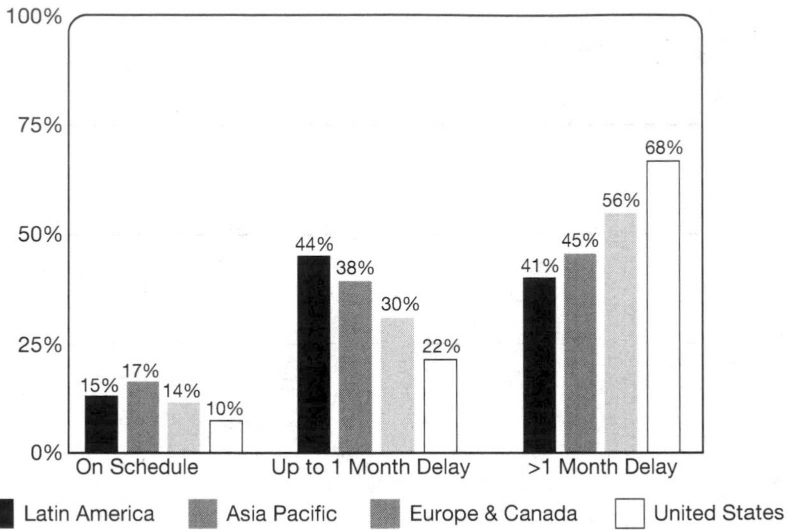

Figure 5-4. Enrollment delays: distribution of delays in site enrollment.
Source: CenterWatch Surveys of U.S. (2009, n=950), Asian (2006, n=156), Latin American (2005, n=317), European and Canadian (2006, n=356) investigative sites.

A manager of a large U.S. study for a midsize sponsor offered a similar comment:

> *I wanted to see why we were losing subjects, and so I asked the CRO for a list of frequency and reasons for screen failures. It took them 11 weeks to produce the list—and then they charged me $1,000 for it!*

Enrollment planning requires a trade-off between the number of sites on the one hand and the cost and complexity of managing them on the other. Regardless of initial plans, however, tracking actual performance is critical.

Facilitating Collection of Enrollment Information

In many cases, enrollment measures become available only when the sponsor or CRO receives CRFs. Studies seldom collect data on the number of individuals screened but found to be ineligible. When studies do collect such data, sites often submit it irregularly or late because of competing priorities. To promote more timely submission of data on enrollment progress, studies should try to make it easy and quick for sites to record and submit relevant information. Integration of data-collection tools with site workflow can help. Today's data software often neglects such issues. The resulting lack of information hobbles both site and study managers.

Tracking Enrollment Progress

Near-real-time data capture and efficient and detailed tracking of enrollment performance can identify patterns in recruitment, referrals, and screen failures, allowing study managers to optimize the enrollment process. Nevertheless, examples of systematic tracking of enrollment strategies are rare in the published literature. Detailed enrollment information often becomes available only after study completion.[3,4] Managing enrollment effectively requires a means of continuously analyzing enrollment performance during the study to determine which sources provide the most patients and which strategies are most successful. Studies should routinely collect, track, and report metrics for individual sites and the study as a whole (see below).

The availability of timely enrollment metrics enables study managers to inform all sites about the strategies in use at high-enrolling sites. The study team can also evaluate study-wide enrollment strategies, including advertising messages and media choices. This detailed, data-driven guidance about potential improvements stands in contrast to the common inability of study managers to know why a site is performing poorly.[5]

KEY ENROLLMENT METRICS

Patients screened

- Number
- Referral source
- Time from referral to initial screening

Patients enrolled

- Number
- Percent of target achieved
- Number active at each stage
- Number completing each study visit or milestone

Frequency and reason for screen failures

Number, reason, and timing of patient dropout and loss to follow-up

Projected dates for last patient in and last patient out

Screening-to-enrollment intervals

Addressing Screen Failures

Timely enrollment metrics allow study management to address a wide range of issues. Screen failures provide a notable example. If a substantial proportion of screen failures relates to a single field of data, there may be an issue in screening procedures or a problem with one or more of the inclusion/exclusion criteria. Inclusion/exclusion criteria are sometimes inflexible for good reason, such as regulatory requirements. However, inclusion/exclusion criteria can also represent arbitrary judgments. It is not unheard of for a study to spend large sums to meet the original criteria when a modest change in one criterion would greatly reduce the study budget without jeopardizing scientific or informational goals.

Recognition of a high proportion of screen failures associated with specific criteria can enable study managers and the sponsor to consider remedial steps. If the maximum age specified for patients is 45 and many otherwise eligible patients are slightly older, sponsors must weigh the relative merits of modestly extending the age criterion versus spending substantially more to meet the original criteria.

The same specific inclusion/exclusion criteria may require rigid treatment in one study and allow greater flexibility in another, depending on considerations such as the way the test drug is metabolized. For example, treating anemia requires patients with a depressed level of hemoglobin. With a drug that is not metabolized hepatically, there may be some leeway on indices of liver function. If numerous patients are screen failing because of marginal liver function, then it makes sense to explore the effects of shifting the cutoff levels of those values. Similarly, for a study of antibiotics, if screen failures are excluding otherwise eligible patients who fall slightly below the 10-gram cutoff for hemoglobin, it may make sense to accept a 9.5-gram level. Only detailed, timely information on reasons for screen failures can provide the opportunity to consider such trade-offs. Although changes in inclusion/exclusion criteria require amending the protocol, the change is often worthwhile if enrollment delays present a serious issue.

Identifying Recruitment Successes

Identifying reasons for successful recruitment is just as important as identifying reasons for screen failures. Recruitment strategies are an area in which operational adaptations can improve results enough to make a real difference in timelines and costs. In many studies, sites try strategies that have worked for them in the past. Some strategies at specific sites may fail and others may quickly yield outstanding results. It is appropriate to identify successful strategies and to encourage all sites, especially those facing the greatest enrollment challenges, to consider adopting them. When remedial efforts fail, study managers may find it necessary to replace underperforming sites with preselected backups.

Reporting Enrollment Information

While some data systems can provide limited information about enrollment progress, few systems in current use provide the level of information essential for truly effective study management. Paper systems are incapable of providing such information. Commercial EDC systems do not collect enrollment information that is timely and detailed enough. Figures 5-5 and 5-6 show data displays from one system that does collect and report this information in real time. The data-capture method, a digital pen, records data immediately in electronic form and allows sites to report enrollment metrics within hours of patient visits. Figure 5-5 shows an information "widget" that provides a high-level summary on a manager's desktop. The display of enrollment metrics receives continuous updates as new data comes in from the field. Figure 5-6 shows a web report that met one sponsor's specific needs for a study involving competitive enrollment.

The central importance of enrollment to study progress justifies providing multiple views of enrollment information, each view providing clues about possible improvements. For example, studies using competitive enrollment need even the most basic reports to allow comparing the performance of different sites. Visual displays such as that shown in Figure 5-6 provide

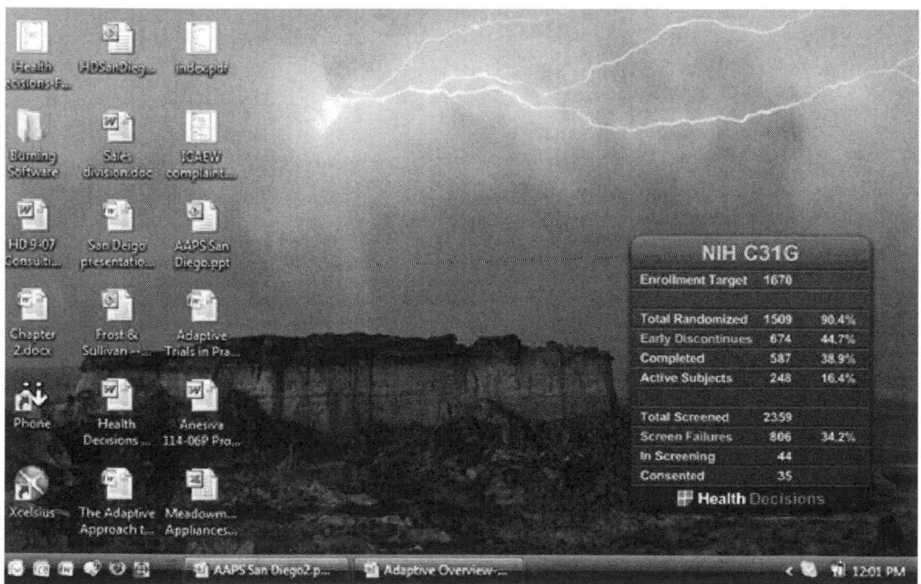

Figure 5-5. Desktop widget provides project summary information. The most useful widgets are specific to each study role; this display shows the project manager's study overview. Data categories hyperlink to a web page containing more extensive information, including data by site and over time.

Source: Health Decisions, Inc. Copyright 2007,

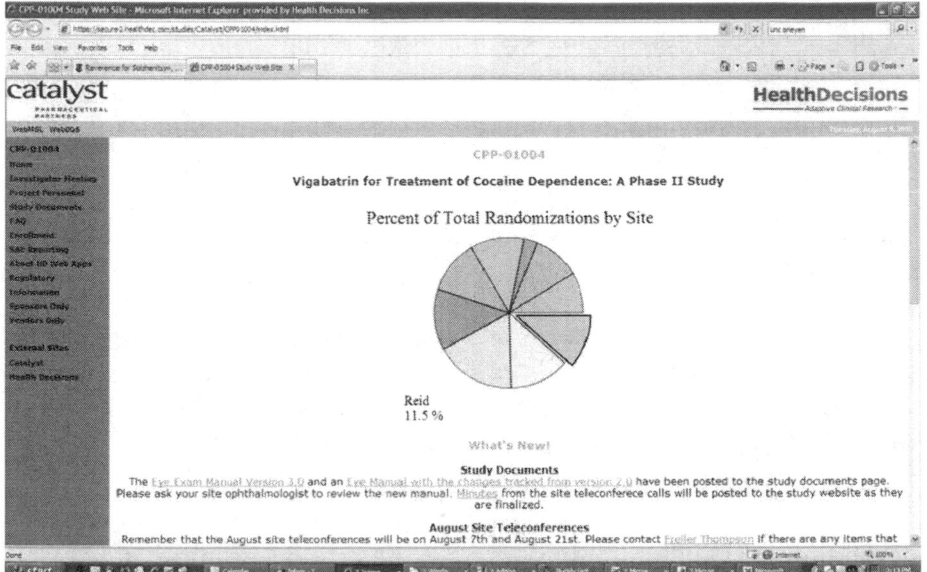

Figure 5-6. A report showing enrollment distribution by site in a study that used competitive enrollment techniques. Mouse rollover highlights individual sites, allowing the study team to determine each site's contribution immediately. Links to supporting pages provide additional information such as number of patients screened and frequency and reasons for screen failure.

Source: Catalyst Pharmaceuticals and Health Decisions, Inc.

a simple, accurate means for a sponsor or site to check site performance. Since enrollment and other factors change while the study is in progress, it is important to be able to make quick changes as to what data is displayed and how.

Example 5-1: Improving slow enrollment

A sponsor initiated two studies of STD treatment using different CROs. One CRO selected a recruitment strategy based on conventional methods. The CRO monitored progress at a typical pace based on receiving updates through monitor visits and calls. Recruitment for the studies centered on selecting six investigational sites likely to have large populations meeting inclusion/exclusion criteria. Recruitment tracking consisted primarily of counts of the number of patients enrolled at each site and in the entire study. Recruitment progress was disappointing. Lacking detailed information, the CRO had no recourse but to add more sites and increase spending on promotion. However, the addition of radio advertisements and three additional sites failed to increase enrollment to the level required.

The second CRO began by selecting six sites much like those selected by the first CRO. However, the second CRO continuously tracked not only numbers of patients screened and enrolled but also details such as reasons for screen failures. Site progress metrics came from either data transmitted as sites completed forms or continuously updated summary information on the study's dedicated website. Initially, the six sites enrolled patients at approximately the same rate, averaging 3.1 patients per site per month, missing the target rate of 5. However, data quickly showed that one site was enrolling patients almost twice as fast as the next best site.

Nothing in the demographics or patterns of screen failures seemed to explain recruitment successes at the high-performing site. The study manager asked the monitor in charge of that site to find out the reason. The site coordinator told the monitor, "I don't know what other sites are doing, but we thought about where individuals at high risk for STD are likely to be found and realized that they probably spend more time in nightclubs than in doctors' offices. So we began discussing posting notices with several nightclubs in the area when the study started. It took a couple of weeks, but after we began posting notices in nightclub bathrooms, our enrollment really took off."

The study manager quickly developed a program encouraging other sites to try the successful recruitment strategy. E-mail linked sites to a web page providing criteria for selecting nightclubs and a downloadable template for a recruitment flyer. The study provided budget for printing and distribution. Most sites adopted the suggestion. Figure 5-7 shows the result. Enrollment increased to 8.1 patients per month.

The study's goal was to enroll 330 patients in 11 months. The study enrolled the desired number of patients in only 9 months. Had the average monthly enrollment remained at 3.1 patients, the study would have taken 18 months—double the time required with the new strategy.

Source: Health Decisions, Inc.

A similar example comes from a study in which one site developed a television advertisement. Close tracking of enrollment figures revealed a sudden jump at the site and simplified identifying the reason for the jump. Study management quickly shared the successful advertising approach with underperforming sites, and enrollment picked up for the entire study.

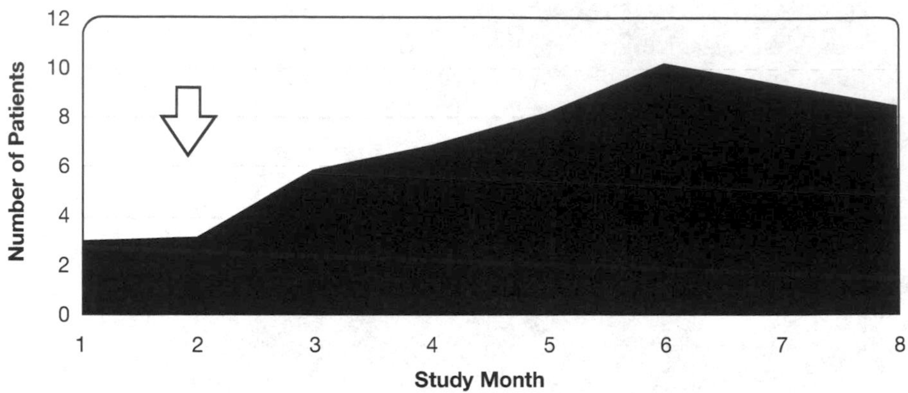

Figure 5-7. Overall enrollment for STD study. After sites began advertising in nightclub restrooms, following the lead of the fastest-enrolling site (arrow), enrollment improved quickly. Close tracking of enrollment and other performance metrics allowed quick identification of the most successful enrollment strategy.
Source: Health Decisions, Inc. Copyright 2003. Used by permission.

Example 5-2: Controlling high screen-failure rate

In a recent study of patients with chronic kidney disease (CKD), the screen-failure rate at all sites substantially exceeded the rate anticipated. Tracking reasons for screen failure traced most failures to two laboratory criteria. Two months after study initiation, the study added two sites and redoubled emphasis on careful patient selection. These changes allowed meeting original enrollment timelines despite the disappointing start.

Source: Health Decisions, Inc.

In another CKD study involving the same product, the CRO was able to identify the need to change withdrawal criteria in a protocol amendment based on timely reporting of subject withdrawal rate and reasons for discontinuation. These interventions saved 4 months off an initial 14-month timeline.
Source: Health Decisions, Inc.

Example 5-3: Modification of inclusion/exclusion criteria

In a study of growth hormone in patients with short stature, study managers noticed that an absolute age cutoff was excluding a high proportion of patients evaluated for the study despite satisfactory maturation indices and height, weight, and laboratory evaluations. With regulatory agreement, the sponsor slightly amended the inclusion criteria to focus on indices of maturation rather than age. The result was a rapid 20% increase in enrollment.

Source: Health Decisions, Inc.

Data Quality

Data quality is of paramount importance, both as an endpoint for clinical studies and because the rework associated with assuring data quality is a major cost. Ensuring data quality requires tracking the numerous study activities that affect the accuracy of data collection and reporting, including forms and related instructions. Equally important is ensuring that site and study personnel have the training necessary to minimize data-entry errors and promote data quality.

Forms and Instructions

While the importance of clear, unambiguous forms and instructions is beyond dispute, many studies discover too late that they have fallen short of this goal. Close data tracking allows determining whether forms and instructions are performing as desired and, if not, where improvements are necessary. For example, if early reports show all sites have a high query rate for a specific CRF field, the reason is very likely a flawed CRF design or inadequate instructions for entering data in the field. It is not always possible to alter forms and instructions during a study, but improved instructions and training can minimize the effect of poorly designed forms and procedures on future studies if not the one in progress.

Data Management/CRFs

The cost for addressing each query is approximately $350.[6] A conventional study of modest size, generating approximately 100,000 data points, typically produces 5,000–10,000 queries. Total costs for resolving queries in such a study would therefore range from $1.75 to $3.5 million. Studies that are larger or more complex can incur much higher costs for data corrections. Indirect costs are appreciable as well. Errors in data can delay achieving milestones such as database locks, whether interim or final. Measures of data quality help identify underlying problems and provide a basis for adaptive management techniques that increase data accuracy and minimize delays.

Study management often treats generating, tracking, and resolving queries—the most fundamental study process—as a necessity with unavoidable costs associated with unalterable procedures. Since managers believe they can do little to change the query process, it receives little scrutiny and may not be clearly defined. The result is confusion about responsibilities and procedures for query handling and a variety of inefficiencies such as duplication of queries. Some companies distribute data from the field internally and allow anybody to generate queries on the same data. A single error can generate multiple queries from different functional areas, leading to redundant efforts on multiple levels. The same query can take on a second life in a version with slightly different wording. Investigators can receive related queries from multiple sources within the same company (ref. 1, p. 152).

Efficient data management requires close tracking of incoming data. For best results, this tracking should be detailed enough to identify which CRFs and questions are causing the most queries and which changes in forms, instructions, procedures, and training can eliminate problems that are causing high query rates. At a minimum, data tracking should include:

- site-specific information;
- query rate by site and by interviewer;
- time from patient visit to data submission;
- time to query response;
- average number of unresolved queries;
- personnel turnover and training requirements (often shared with clinical departments);
- feedback on whether the CRF facilitates or interferes with site workflow;
- overall study figures for above metrics.

Example 5-4: Early identification and correction of site personnel issues

A global assessment of an Alzheimer's disease product involves complex assessments of cognitive function through several standardized tests requiring administration by trained professionals. In one such study, study managers were watching the data as it accumulated and noticed a sudden change in one of the outcome measures. Although the individual responses fell within the prescribed range and did not trigger a query, the recent responses differed quite a bit from previous measurements. A closer look at the performance of other subjects for the site and a number of general performance measures suggested that something had happened to diminish the quality of the site's work, but the discordant study responses were of particular concern because study managers realized that each individual represented a considerable investment as well as that additional variance in response measurements would diminish the statistical power.

Although the site monitor that called the site did not receive any specific responses that indicated a problem, there were enough vague issues that she decided on an early monitoring visit. That visit quickly revealed the source of at least several of the problems: the tester certified and trained at the initial investigator meeting was on medical leave, and an untrained individual was administering the cognitive assessments. Although the site had good intentions, the suspect results required, after lengthy discussions with the medical monitor, reassessments in some cases and elimination of one subject from the study. In addition, two patients who had recently been admitted were found to be ineligible and were discontinued. Early discovery of these errors allowed intervention before expenditure of additional money on excluded patients. Intervention also reduced the risk of compromising study results.

Source: Health Decisions, Inc.

Improving Data Precision

Data variability is a key measure of the quality of data collected. Data precision varies inversely with variability. Thus, the more precise the data, the smaller the study required to demonstrate a given effect. Greater-than-planned variability can quickly undermine a study's ability to detect a difference between a drug and its comparator. Demonstrating a given effect may require a larger sample size. Controlling variability is a key goal of the agile approach to study management. Measures of data quality such as query rates and rapid feedback on errors enable interventions that limit variability. The quality of study data and the quality of study management thus go hand in hand.

Minimizing data variability has paramount importance in certain therapeutic areas that rely on subjective outcome measures. Central nervous system (CNS) outcomes are a prime example. The subjective outcome measures are so variable that things like the amount of sleep a subject got the previous night can affect outcome measures. Alzheimer's studies confront this problem since they involve neuropsychological testing to assess memory and cognitive ability. Studies take pains to use standardized tests, each with its own internal measure of variance, and to have carefully trained evaluators administer tests consistently in order to minimize extraneous variability. In such studies, minimizing data variability is critically important to controlling study power, size, and, ultimately, cost and duration. An increase of 50% in variability of ADAS-cog, a questionnaire used in studies of Alzheimer's treatments, can increase sample size from 81 to 180 in each of two arms, an increase of 200 in the number of patients needed for a study. Extensive performance metrics and the ability to carry out operational adaptations can greatly reduce the variability of data. Evaluating variability during the course of a study also allows compensating for greater-than-planned variability through sample-size reestimation, as described in Chapter 4.

Monitoring

Site monitors are both vital and expensive. Monitoring costs account for about one-third of study budgets. Effective steps to reduce monitoring costs include replacing error-prone manual processes with electronic tools and allocating monitoring attention based on field measurements of quality and quantity. The usual practice calls for rigid adherence to monitoring intervals established at the beginning of each study, sometimes before sites have generated data.

Adaptive Allocation of Monitoring Effort

Continuous tracking of number of unverified fields at each site allows allocating site visits according to need rather than an arbitrary schedule. This keeps data monitoring up to date and eliminates unnecessary and premature visits. Toward the end of a study, metrics such as those tracking unverified source fields help prevent delays in database lock. Use of such metrics has helped reduce one CRO's average lock times to 10 days for most studies (Health Decisions, Inc.).

For a confirmatory study of a drug for prostate cancer, an adaptive approach relied on measures of the quantity and quality of data generated at each site. The adaptive approach in this instance determined monitoring frequency for each site based on the number of unmonitored fields at the site and an index of data quality that included number and rate of queries and patterns of questions that generated queries. This information allowed monitors to determine what was causing queries and to address root causes early on. The net benefit was reducing the number of monitoring visits to approximately one-half the number expected under a conventional fixed-interval monitoring schedule.

Example 5-5: Adaptive monitoring

Planners estimated that an oncology study would require 2.5 years for field data collection, 100 sites, and monitoring visits to each site at eight-week intervals. Costs involved included $80/hr for monitors (fully burdened), travel cost per visit of $600, and an average of 32 hours per interim monitoring visit. A conventional monitoring approach with the same component costs would involve 1,625 visits and 52,000 monitor hours, with costs of $4,160,000 for labor and

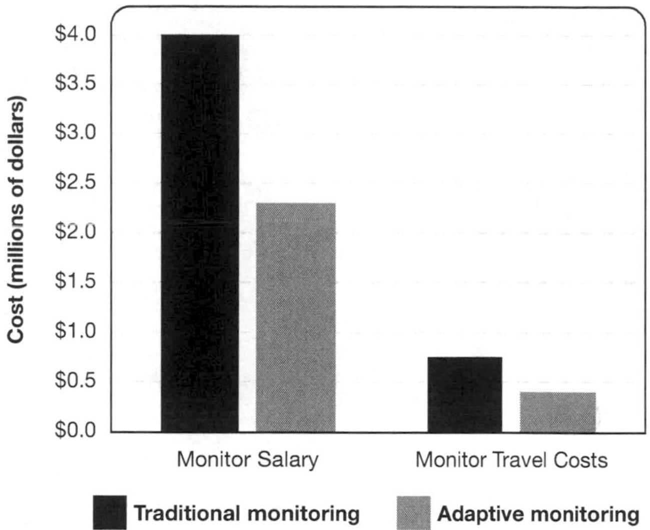

Figure 5-8. Comparative cost for travel and monitor time using conventional and adaptive monitoring.

$975,000 for travel, for a total monitoring cost of $5.135 million. The study included 1,000,000 data fields. Study managers estimated each individual monitor's ability to source-verify fields, using electronic monitoring tools, at 1,000 per day. (For more on electronic monitoring tools, see below, "The Transformative Role of Technology.") Applying these estimates to the figures in the previous paragraph, the adaptive approach involved 1,000 interim monitoring visits, each taking 32 hours. The total was thus 32,000 hours for monitoring at a cost of $2.56 million and $600,000 travel costs, for a total of $3.16 million. The net savings compared to the conventional approach was $1.975 million, or 38% (Figure 5-8).

A Flexible Team Approach to Monitoring

The standard practice in monitoring clinical studies is to specify a monitoring plan at the outset and stick to it. The main elements of a monitoring plan are monitoring procedures that emphasize site visits, assignment of specific sites to each monitor, and monitoring intervals that are the same for all sites. Barring staff turnover, the initial plan remains the same throughout the study.

The previous section of this chapter described adaptive allocation of site visits based on the need for visits rather than fixed intervals. Maximizing the efficiency of monitoring activities requires adapting other aspects of monitoring based on evolving conditions during the study. Workload at each site in actual studies does not always match initial assignments. Monitoring tasks vary in complexity and urgency at different times at all sites. Modern computers and communications allow performing some monitoring tasks from a central office rather than on site. With so many variables in play, monitoring is best viewed as a dynamic, team-based activity that adapts as necessary to actual circumstances during a study.

One important way to improve monitoring efficiency is to assess the need for a monitor on site to perform each task. The ability to review and verify data in-house shortly after patient visits opens new possibilities. Provided there is access to current data and site performance metrics based on timely data collection, monitors can address many queries and other issues at their sites from the home office between site visits.

Monitoring effort should also adapt by matching the capabilities of individuals with the volume, complexity, and urgency of monitoring tasks at each site. Whether performed on site or in a central office, different monitoring tasks require different capabilities. Clinical trials assistants can provide support for more senior monitoring personnel and help with detailed work that includes tracking incoming data and performance metrics to detect issues before they can develop into problems. Junior monitors can perform most routine monitoring tasks, managing an average load of perhaps seven to eight sites. Senior monitors can contribute flexibly, monitoring some sites and overseeing less experienced monitors, reviewing visit reports, and performing other higher-level tasks as necessary. Finally, monitors sometimes encounter problems that demand the attention of the project manager. As a rule of thumb, one to four clinical trials assistants will support each traveling monitor and the project manager.

Monitors must still visit sites, but they can do much of their work by telephone and e-mail, reducing the need for travel. Monitors maintain regular site contacts, follow up on in-house issues, assist with regular query resolution, attend regular team meetings, and take part in periodic training. The result of the dynamic, team-based approach is faster, higher quality work. This approach also offers monitors a more appealing work environment and less travel, bolstering retention rates and improving long-term performance.

The Transformative Role of Technology

Studies can improve efficiency not only by dynamically allocating the effort of monitors, but also by improving the efficiency of the activity of monitoring itself. The role of the site monitor evolved primarily as a means of ensuring the accuracy of collected data and adherence to study procedures. While at investigational sites, monitors spend most of their time

KEY SITE-MONITORING METRICS

Query rate

Queries outstanding

Time to resolve queries

Fields, forms, and edit checks (normal ranges) generating most queries

Cumulative number of unmonitored fields

GCP compliance

Protocol violations

Adverse events

Serious adverse events

laboriously checking the data collected by the study against corresponding data where first written. Patient charts usually contain this source data. Monitors hand check stacks of paper printouts of database values against medical records. Monitors note discrepancies with sticky notes and jot queries by hand without benefit of templates or computer assistance. In sum, monitors slave away at a tedious, expensive, manual process. As with any manual task, the work of monitors has high error rates.

While there are numerous issues in work that monitors do, the biggest issue is what they have no time to do. Monitors can rarely look up from the tedious proofreading, box-checking process to consider site management. The focus on identifying and correcting individual errors leaves little time for searching out patterns of problems and taking action to prevent recurrences. Monitors seldom enjoy the luxury of thinking about how to optimize site performance and increase the likelihood of a successful study. Particularly adept monitors may take the initiative and consider the bigger picture. However, recruitment of monitors seldom considers managerial capacity, and the constant focus on minutiae impairs development of higher-level skills.

Monitor as Manager

A more productive approach to monitoring leaves repetitive, rote tasks to machines that do them faster, freeing up humans to concentrate on what they do better than machines—managing. Electronic tools enable a comprehensive data management approach that allows for timely CRF data import as well as query resolution on an ongoing basis between monitoring visits.[7] This new approach to monitoring becomes possible because of the availability of current metrics providing reliable insight into site performance, including the likely sources of recurrent problems. Monitors can concentrate on ensuring high levels of site performance by diagnosing and addressing each site's unique issues. Monitors can also identify and address emerging problems before they become a significant drain on study resources. Early intervention greatly reduces the amount of rework required to maintain high data quality.

Technology and Basic Monitoring Tasks

Recently developed technological tools allow electronic checking of database values against source documents.[7] Truly electronic data-capture methods—methods that allow electronic records to serve as source documentation—provide striking advances in monitoring efficiency. Since verifying information from the study database against paper versions of source documents can consume 80% or more of monitoring effort, the ability to ensure data accuracy without such extensive reliance on highly trained and compensated staff could provide great savings. One-third of a typical study budget goes to source data verification. Operational adaptations can reduce the workload for source-verification activities by 80%, resulting in savings of $2.6 million on a $10 million study. Electronic tools make such a reduction attainable.

Good clinical practices (GCP) standards define source data as the initial recording of a piece of information. In most cases, since site personnel first record information in patient records, those records are the source data. Sites complete CRFs by copying data from these source records. Even web-EDC systems typically use an intermediate worksheet to record this information before manual entry at a computer. However, newer data-capture methods can allow first recording patient data in electronic form, making this the source data.

The digital pen is one data-capture technology that meets regulatory requirements for electronic source documents. (For more on the digital pen, see Chapter 9, "The Agile Platform.") With regulatory acceptance, studies have used electronic data captured by the digital pen as source material. This is most common with smaller safety studies, especially when subjects do not have previous medical charts. In other instances, when paper patient charts and electronic study CRFs must contain the same information, data capture by digital pen satisfies this need in a straightforward manner. When the study management system receives the data, it reformats the data immediately for inclusion in a site's patient chart and then transmits the reformatted electronic data back to sites. The sites can then print out the reformatted data and paste it into the patient's records. This approach allows storage of the electronic source document, the CRF, at a central location while the site retains a copy for archiving. The electronic copy includes a time and date stamp for each pen stroke, an unalterable record of original documentation. An electronic query system provides the only mechanism for data updates. This system includes an audit trail that verifies changes through printed copies signed by the investigator.

Redefining Work Processes

Capture of electronic source data exemplifies how technology allows redefining existing processes to make them faster, more accurate, and less expensive. This approach makes data immediately available to study managers. The process of checking data can begin within minutes of a site's first recording the data. Sites can submit data upon completion of each CRF. In contrast, conventional practice allows study CRFs to remain at a site for weeks before a monitor performs a manual check. The approach using electronic data as source greatly improves on the conventional practice of leaving paper CRFs at each site until a monitor can review data manually and then returning paper CRFs to a central location for data entry and the beginning of electronic validation. The latter approach effectively hobbles any attempt at adaptive decision making, whether for design or operational adaptations.

While the potential use of electronic medical records (EMRs) as source documents is appealing, this is not yet a practical possibility. To begin with, typical medical records and CRFs have served different purposes and have different requirements. Before EMRs can serve as source, the specific EMR system must undergo validation for research under Title 21 Code of Federal Regulations Part 11 (21 CFR Part 11), which governs electronic systems used in clinical trials.[8] There are also confidentiality issues to resolve. With greater standardization in how EMR systems handle data, such as use of Extensisble Markup Language (XML) tags, the use of EMRs as source data will gain momentum. However, it will take years for medical institutions to complete the transition to EMRs. Thus, it will be quite some time before EMRs establish themselves as standard source documents for clinical studies.

However, electronic tools can already provide considerable improvements in the efficiency of source document verification. A monitor can bring an electronic copy of the database to the site for quicker comparison of each value with patient records or other source material. The electronic tool simplifies issuing prompt queries to resolve discrepancies. In practice, the use of this tool has allowed field monitors to verify twice as many fields per hour as previous methods. If monitoring accounts for one-third of the cost of a study, and source verification consumes 80% of a monitor's time, then this tool can save about $1.3 million on a $10 million study.

Site Closeout and Database Lock

In a sense, the overriding purpose of adaptive monitoring from study inception is to pave the way for quick, efficient, and trouble-free site closeout and database lock. Monitors can consider the likely effect on site closeout and database lock of all events from the outset of the study. By focusing on issues with the potential to complicate site closeout, monitors can minimize potential delays in the critical last weeks of the study. With conventional monitoring and paper source data, surprises in the data can appear very late, complicating database lock and perhaps even data analysis. Adaptive monitoring minimizes the possibility of late, unpleasant surprises.

In effect, site closeout strategy should begin at study startup. That is the time to implement the most important single measure to ensure efficient site closeout: timely data capture, cleaning, and validation. Timely availability of performance metrics allows monitors and study managers to identify problems with the potential to complicate the later stages of a trial. If cleaning, validation and verification against source materials have long been complete, and if the study team has identified, understood, and addressed problems as they emerged, then site closeout will be routine and quick. Conversely, if numerous unresolved queries are still lingering at the end of a study, site closeout can become a nightmare for monitors.

Incremental Site Closeout

To maximize efficiency, monitors should close out each site not in one large batch but by individual patient. This ensures the earliest identification of any remaining problems and the greatest opportunity to resolve them. Rather than waiting for completion of data on the last patient at each site before initiating closeout, monitors should push to close out one patient at a time and as early as possible. This obviously reduces the amount of work that remains in the crucial period when timelines grow short and anxiety high. If a surprising event affects data on a patient that the study has already closed out, the study can reopen data on that patient.

The interval between the last patient's last visit (LPLV) and database lock is one of the most intensely watched intervals in clinical research. Following database lock, analysis will pronounce the verdict on months or years of work. Therefore, everyone involved in the study is eager to minimize the interval between LPLV and database lock. The methodical observation of basic adaptive principles during and particularly towards the end of each study can reduce this interval from months to weeks or weeks to days. Barring any complicating factors such as last-minute severe adverse outcomes, which must generally be followed up for 30 days after occurrence, a study can take several steps to accelerate database lock. The purpose of the steps is to minimize the amount of work required in the study's last week or two. Such steps include:

- progressive lock of CRF, visit, and patient;
- staggered visits during the study, with emphasis on early database lock;
- tracking of number of unmonitored fields and other critical-path site activities;
- allocating adequate personnel for rapid data validation and query resolution.

With careful planning, rigorous execution, optimized processes, and electronic tools, much faster closeout becomes an attainable goal. This same improved process for study closeout also facilitates rapid database lock for interim assessments for objectives such as sample-size reestimation.

Example 5-6: Adaptive site closeout, forecasting closeout dates, one patient at a time

When a sponsor learned that a company with a competing product intended to announce the results of a major study earlier than anticipated, the sponsor decided to accelerate preliminary database lock and interim analysis by six weeks. The large and complex oncology study involved eight sites in the United States.

Usual industry practice would attempt to meet the sudden requirement with brute force—more money and more people to divide the workload. In this case, two different CROs were conducting similar companion studies. The first CRO announced that its standard operating procedures (SOPs) did not allow locking the database six weeks early—it was impossible. The sponsor pressed, offering to pay for extra workers. The CRO indicated that even with more personnel, it would be impossible to complete the necessary work in the allotted time.

The second CRO utilized detailed status and performance tracking indices in managing the study. This CRO used such performance measures to assess the effort required for early database lock. The first step was determining how much work remained at each site and in the aggregate. As Table 5-1 shows, the amount of work remaining varied greatly by site. Sites had between 0 and 6,028 unverified fields.

Table 5-1. Work remaining at each of eight sites to close out a large study.

Site	Subjects With Data	Total Fields	Verified Fields	Unverified Fields	Percent Verified
101	1	695	667	28	96.0
102	5	2,853	1,582	1,271	55.5
104	2	1,554	1,554	0	100.0
105	12	11,327	5,299	6,028	46.8
106	3	1,200	9	1,191	0.8
107	1	618	597	21	96.6
110	4	3,367	2,867	500	85.1
113	3	1,627	1,328	299	81.6
TOTAL	**31**	**23,241**	**13,903**	**9,338**	**59.8**

Based on a 3% query rate, study managers expected source-data verification (SDV) to generate an additional 280 queries, for a total of 9,618 data items to verify on site. Managers estimated the remaining number of required site visits and time needed per visit based on monitors' daily field verification rates. Since the seven monitors had verified an average of 647 fields per day, or about 92 each, managers calculated that about 15 days of work remained (Table 5-2). They assigned four monitors to complete work at site 105, one at site 102, one at site 106, and one to start at site 110 and move to the nearest remaining site. The CRO completed database lock two days early.

Table 5-2. Estimated number of onsite monitoring days required for database lock.

Site	Estimated Total Data to Monitor	Estimated No. of Onsite Days for SDV
101	28	0.04
102	1271	1.96
104	0	0.00
105	6028	9.32
106	1191	1.84
107	21	0.03
110	500	0.77
113	299	0.46
Follow-up	280	0.43
TOTAL	**9,618**	**14.87**

Supporting Functions for Efficient Operations

Adaptive studies depend on efficient study-wide communications, laboratory work, and supply management. Breakdowns in any of these areas can prevent studies from realizing the benefits of adaptive methods.

Communications

Conducting an adaptive study requires the ability to share a broad range of information quickly and effectively. Communications play an essential role not only in rapid data collection and cleaning but also in implementing corrective measures.

Study Website

The study should make all documents, forms, and training materials available electronically for convenient access by all sites. A simple way to achieve this goal is to create a custom study website providing all study documents and continuously updated performance metrics. Password protection restricts access based on study role and need to know. Reports showing mean or comparative site performance allow sites to compare their performance with peers. Comparative performance information not only informs sites but also motivates them.

Primary functions of a study website include:

- ensuring that all sites have access to the most recent and complete study documents;
- keeping all sites informed of progress at other sites;
- providing information on the most successful strategies adopted at different sites;
- encouraging sites to share information on both problems and successes;
- quickly alerting all sites to emerging problems;
- providing information on study progress as individually appropriate for everyone involved.

By providing such information, the study website allows individual sites and investigators to reflect on their own performance and address issues that may have escaped the attention of monitors and study managers. There is often great expertise distributed across the many sites participating in a study. However, it is difficult to harness distributed expertise to benefit the study as a whole. The website brings distributed expertise into play. While dedicated study managers will probably provide most insights, an appropriate outlet allows investigators to contribute invaluable observations. Investigators can also adapt their own performance based on the latest information. A good study website affords investigators such opportunities.

Communications for Safety Monitoring

Immediate access to data provides a timely perspective on a variety of safety issues. This is more critical in early testing but remains vital throughout development and into the postmarketing arena. Use of data-collection tools that allow continuous monitoring of safety reports represents a big advance over the batch-and-queue method that currently predominates. Continuous tracking of safety information is desirable because definitions of safety endpoints are generally less specific than definitions of efficacy measures. The "soft" nature of many safety endpoints increases the need for ongoing assessment relative to historical controls, a comparator, or even a subjective impression.

The immediacy of safety reporting is perhaps nowhere more important than in early drug testing, when dose advancement depends on the safety parameters from each dose. For dose-escalation studies, for example, the decision to increase dose for the next cohort depends on having data for the current cohort. Immediate methods of data acquisition can substantially ease this task. Figure 6-2 (next chapter) shows a data display of a phase I study in which the sponsor has access to safety data an average of four hours after the safety observation period closes. The site interviews each patient at the end of the period and docks a digital pen to upload data electronically. Data management procedures automatically sort and display the data. This approach reduces decision cycles from the usual one or two weeks to a single day.

Reporting and Assessing Laboratory Results

Laboratory studies play indispensible roles in almost all studies, whether focused on safety or efficacy. Study managers should consider closely monitoring lab performance. This is particularly true early in a study and for tests that involve specialized areas. Inaccurate lab results can undermine an otherwise exemplary study. This concern merits special attention in areas where even specialized labs may have limited experience and perform relatively few evaluations. Endocrinology studies provide one example. Electronic receipt of laboratory values simplifies the use of automated reports to identify out-of-range lab results. Reports that flag out-of-range results allow quick intervention.

Example 5-7: Assessing lab results

During the early phase of a pediatric study of growth hormone, far more children than anticipated had exclusionary insulinlike growth factor 1 (IGF-1) results. Values for IGF-1 collected at screening were within range at the time of screening, yet the results for the first follow-up were frequently out of range. After repeated prompting, the sponsor contacted the lab. The lab discovered that the specialized lab assay had drifted out of calibration without detection, causing spurious results.

Supply-Chain Management

The increasing complexity of trials, greater geographic diversity, and added demands of adaptive trials increase the need for effective supply-chain management. The days of ordering drugs once and tracking supplies by spreadsheet are over. Supply-chain management must now support fast-moving studies that may shift patients, dosing, and sites.

Operational challenges require electronic systems to track supplies, with on-hand levels decremented at the time of enrollment. The main adaptive

RULES FOR OPERATIONAL ADAPTATIONS

- *Everyone on the study team must accept the concept of adapting throughout a study.*
- *Study startup requires aggressive timelines, early identification of problems at investigational sites, and prompt resort to backup strategies, such as reserve sites, to prevent delays.*
- *Data cleaning should begin with data capture.*
- *Data is not truly captured until it enters the study database.*
- *Data must be quickly converted to both knowledge and metaknowledge—performance metrics.*
- *Decisions based on knowledge and metaknowledge from current trial data are the only way to make successful operational adaptations.*
- *Monitors must adapt their schedules based on site performance metrics and focus attention based on need rather than rigid schedules.*
- *Steps to facilitate site closeout should begin with study startup, including prompt data cleaning and query resolution.*
- *Site closeout should proceed progressively rather than addressing one site at a time.*

change is adjusting the level of resupply of drugs and comparators, given fixed constraints such as time required for production and packaging.

An adaptive trial may evaluate a range of doses that are difficult to predict and therefore to stockpile. Suppose early dose-finding studies involve doses from 10 to 400 mg, with little sense of which doses will prove most successful. Such a study might involve 10- and 50-mg capsules. An adaptive platform provides the ability to move straight into phase III immediately after reducing the number of dosing arms to the number desired for confirmatory testing. However, the supply chain may constrain the transition. Suppose the smallest pill contains 10 mg and the largest 50 mg but the dose selected for confirmatory testing is 200 or 300 mg. Studies prefer not to require patients to take the number of tablets required to provide the desired doses using the supplies ordered for dose finding. Study managers face a potentially difficult choice between moving directly into the confirmatory phase and halting operations to arrange for a more convenient 100-mg tablet.

A platform that simplifies predicting future dose requirements based on historical data is particularly valuable in adaptive studies. Projections based on knowledge of early response may allow greater lead time for manufacturing, packaging, printing, or other study needs.

The Bottom Line

This chapter has shown how operational adaptations allow study managers to achieve greater efficiency by responding quickly to changing information about key study activities. This approach to management exemplifies agile clinical development.

The next chapter explores the ways in which design and operational adaptations can work together to maximize efficiency. The combination of design and operational adaptations and the infrastructure and processes required to support them can and should modernize clinical research. Pharma companies already devote enormous human, material, and scientific resources to clinical development. The agile approach to clinical development can put these resources to far more productive use.

References

1 Streamlining clinical trials. Durham, NC: Cutting Edge Information; 2008.

2 CenterWatch Surveys of U.S. (2009, *n*=950), Asian (2006, *n*=156), Latin American (2005, *n*=317), European and Canadian (2006, n=356) investigative sites.

3 Galbreath AD, Smith B, Wood P, Forkner E, Peters JI. Cumulative recruitment experience in two large single-center, randomized controlled clinical trials. Contemp Clin Trials. 2008;29:335–42.

4 Sweet S, Legro RS, Coney P. A comparison of methods and results in recruiting white and black women into reproductive studies: the MMC-PSIIU cooperating center on reproduction experience. Contemp Clin Trials. 2008;29:478–81.

5 Monaghan H, et al. A randomised trial of the effects of an additional communication strategy on recruitment into a large, multi-centre trial. Contemp Clin Trials. 2007;28(1):1–5.

6 Malakoff D. Spiraling costs threaten gridlock. Science. 2008;322:210–3.

7 Borfitz D. Decisions, decisions: Michael Rosenberg on adaptive research. Bio-ITWorld's eCliniqua newsletter. Sept 6, 2007. Available from: http://www.bio-itworld.com/newsitems/2007/sept/09-06-07-rosenberg.

8 U.S. Department of Health and Human Services, Food and Drug Administration, Center for Drug Evaluation and Research (CDER). Washington. Guidance for Industry. Part 11, Electronic Records; Electronic Signatures — Scope and Application. Aug 2003. Available from: http://www.fda.gov/cder/guidance/5667fnl.htm.

— Chapter 6 —

Agile Clinical Development

Previous chapters show how individual design adaptations and operational adaptations can separately speed development programs and improve efficiency. When design and operational adaptations work in concert on multiple levels, the benefits ripple through every aspect of development. With appropriate technological infrastructure and optimized work processes, studies gain the ability to evaluate study progress continuously and comprehensively. Studies can adapt as circumstances change and problems emerge. Even in the absence of overt problems, studies can improve operations continuously. Agile clinical development best denotes the powerful combination of continuous assessment and refinement with the ability to adapt both design and operations.

The agile approach provides both high velocity and high efficiency in clinical research. Daily activities focus on ensuring the availability of timely information to support decisions that optimize everything from field tasks to design. Achieving such comprehensive optimization requires infrastructure that provides a continuous stream of timely information and simplifies interpretation through flexible reporting and ease of use. Chapter 9, "The Agile Platform," describes the platform in detail. In broad terms, the infrastructure must provide information as appropriate and necessary to support tasks assigned to people in a variety of study roles. This enabling technology platform is essential for any study that hopes to realize the benefits of adaptive methods or the agile approach. Optimized work processes based on lean principles support a systematic effort to make the most effective possible use of time and resources.

A major benefit of agile development is the ability to select and incorporate specific design and operational adaptations as appropriate. Based on the

The Agile Approach to Adaptive Research, by Michael J. Rosenberg needs of any specific study, the agile approach may employ a single design adaptation, more than one, or none. On the other hand, most operational adaptations can contribute to virtually all studies. The degree of emphasis on each operational area depends on the expected level of difficulty in achieving associated goals.

Benefits of Agile Development

Agile development improves the efficiency of clinical studies by enabling superior capabilities in several areas, including:

- **Control:** Availability of accurate, actionable data enables rapid decision making on all levels, resulting in superior control of study activities.
- **Transparency:** The agile approach allows team members to see information relevant to each person's assigned tasks and, subject to blinding limitations, to see whatever other information they want to see, when they want to see it.
- **Risk management:** Since the agile approach allows quick detection of suboptimal performance and identification of causes, it allows prompt action to contain risk and implement contingency plans.
- **Distributed workload:** Through such features as flexible reporting appropriate for each study role and study-wide access to current information, the agile approach allows distributing workload optimally between a central office and the field; an in-house team can perform many tasks traditionally done at high cost in the field, completing work earlier and reducing travel expenses.
- **Waste and rework reduction:** Since the agile approach focuses on identifying problems and their causes quickly, study management can eliminate the problems that are causing errors, minimizing recurrences rather than tolerating errors and fixing them later.
- **Process refinement:** Rapid, continuous reporting of progress in many study activities allows continuous improvement through corrective actions, additional feedback, and further optimizations as necessary; resolving even small problems early greatly improves efficiency over the life of a study.

A Development Example

The remainder of this chapter provides a series of examples organized around the path that a hypothetical product might take from first safety testing through development and up to market registration. The scenario shows how an optimally planned and executed program could take full advantage of adaptive techniques, supporting infrastructure, and optimized processes—the cornerstones of agile clinical development. No hypothetical development program could capture all the elements and nuances of the enormous variety of development programs across the industry. However, the hypothetical program described shows the power of the agile approach to improve the efficiency of entire programs through the combined use of a variety of enhancements. To the author's knowledge, while many studies have used one or more of the techniques described, no single development program to date has used them in combination through all phases of development. Thus, only a hypothetical program can show the full power of the agile approach to enhance entire programs. The author's hope is that this hypothetical program will suggest ways that program managers can address their specific problems and challenges.

While hypothetical, the example draws on real-world knowledge and experience. The example borrows many elements of programs with which the author has close familiarity. The author believes that the hypothetical program described is no pipedream. It represents a reasonable example of a program designed to maximize the benefits of the agile approach.

Providing such a comprehensive example does not imply that realizing the benefits of agile development requires applying agile principles to every facet of every phase of development. Indeed, Chapters 3, 4, and 5 provide examples of achieving substantial benefits from use of a single technique in a single study. Furthermore, the prudent way to adopt the agile approach is incrementally.

One of the potential benefits of agile clinical development is blurring the lines separating conventional phases of development through techniques such as seamless phase II/III designs. Nevertheless, the conventional development vocabulary referencing separate phases conveniently identifies the chief objectives at different stages in the development cycle, namely early safety testing, dose exploration, and confirmatory testing. This chapter sometimes uses the familiar phase designations to identify the focus of work rather than separate studies or periods.

The drug making its way through development in the following scenario is an orally administered receptor modulator for treatment of a non-life-threatening condition. The indication has relatively short-term clinical outcomes. Available techniques allow measuring clinical response within four weeks. In addition, the scenario assumes the existence of immunologic markers that predict clinical response. However, the markers lack conclusive validation and have yet to win acceptance from regulatory authorities as a surrogate for outcomes in clinical studies.

Program Planning

From the outset, this program aims to accelerate development by taking advantage of design adaptations and operational refinements wherever appropriate. Initial planning involves laying out an entire program, from initial safety studies through proof-of-concept, dose-finding, and confirmatory trials. Transitions between development phases are to be seamless.

The program focuses from the beginning on meeting regulatory requirements for this class of drugs, as defined both in guidance documents and in regulatory discussions. To simplify transitions between phases of development, the program uses the same assessments throughout the life of the program. To the greatest extent possible, the same approach defines outcomes assessed, tools for measuring outcomes, and operational details such as designing a single CRF for continued use through all phases of development. To achieve this goal, planners start with requirements for final approval and work backward.

The program relies on the principles of agile clinical development to realize the goal of conducting a seamless program that begins with safety testing and ends by meeting the goals of confirmatory studies. At each step, tracking and adjustment of key design features as well as numerous aspects of clinical operations allow executing the integrated program schematically represented in Figure 6-1.

To realize such a program, initial planning must devote careful thought to how the sponsor envisions marketing the drug. A key comparator is an injection product already on the market. This approved product's development and regulatory history define a reasonably clear path to regulatory approval for the test drug. From a business development perspective, a central question is whether the new therapeutic agent can demonstrate superiority to the comparator or only noninferiority. The sponsor projects very different revenues and profits for the two possibilities:

Hypothesis	Revenue (millions)	Profit (millions)
Superior to marketed drug	6,000	2,000
Equivalent to marketed drug	3,000	800

Early program planning establishes primary and secondary goals for each phase of development, including, where possible, the program's strategic goals. Planners establish goals for both design and operational aspects of the program (Table 6-1) and identify capabilities required to support these goals. Planners also formulate a variety of plans to address different contingencies.

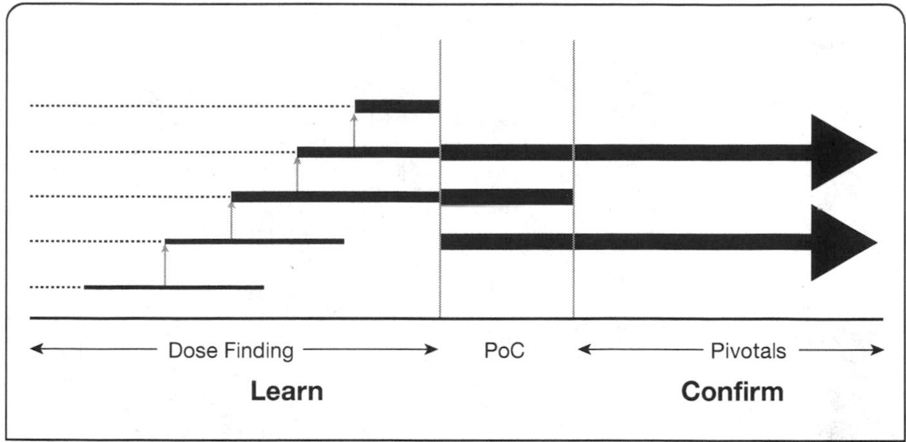

Figure 6-1. Schematic of integrated phase I-II-III agile development program. Line thickness is proportional to cohort size; vertical gray lines represent nominal divisions between activities corresponding to the phases of conventional development programs. In this integrated program, development proceeds seamlessly based on progressive learning from safety testing through confirmatory activities.

Safety Testing (Phase I)

Design

Because the indication is not life threatening and the investigational drug involves a relatively quick response, the strategy for early testing retains a primary focus on safety but also measures the efficacy of both clinical and surrogate outcomes. The sponsor hopes to demonstrate a correlation between the surrogate and clinical outcomes to justify using the surrogates in later development, including confirmatory testing. Early discussions with regulators indicate willingness to consider allowing surrogates in confirmatory testing if earlier testing shows a strong correlation. The ability to use surrogate measures in confirmatory testing would reduce study duration by two to three months, reduce costs, and allow the new product to generate revenue earlier.

The safety evaluation focuses on a four-day response period, an interval largely based on experience with similar products. Study planners decide to use an adaptive dose-finding method rather than gradual, stepwise 3+3 dose escalation from an extremely low dose. The CRM starts with an estimated dose-response curve. In this instance, animal experience with this compound and clinical experience with related compounds provide the basis for defining the curve. The study starts conservatively with a dose about one-third of the curve's maximum value. The study doses a subject at day 0 and collects safety data for four days to aid in determining the

Table 6-1. Goals for program, by phase, including both strategic (light-gray boxes) and operational.

	Primary	Secondary
Safety testing	• Establish MTD • Narrow manufacturing doses	• Efficacy evaluation
	• Decision cycles <4 days • Determine number of sites for next phase	• Pilot study systems, multisite capability • Identify and background work for dose-finding sites • Rapid transition to next phase
Dose finding	• Proof of concept • Select comparator • Assess surrogate • Determine superiority or noninferiority claim • Narrow dosing to < 2 arms • Sample size reestimation at half and three-quarters through study	• Establish study procedures, technology for confirmatory • Lock database, results to FDA <1 month after LPLV • Initiate confirmatory studies <2 months after LPLV
	• Finalize details for confirmatory operations, including drug distribution • Initiate discussions with European regulatory authorities	• Test multicenter project and data management • Initiate European sites, logistics
Confirmatory	• Establish efficacy, safety • Cut 1 treatment arm	• Define target subsets
	• Initiate study within 2 months • Database lock <1 month after LPLV	• Sites in U.S. + Europe • 4-month retention rate >75%
Regulatory	• Submission in <2.5 months after LPLV in confirmatory testing	• Study team in place at LPLV for confirmatory testing -1 month.
	• Table shells complete at LPLV +2 weeks • Draft submission ready at LPLV + 2 weeks	• Document management system fully functional

Note: Detailed lists of supporting elements and contingency plans stemmed from this basic list.

next dose. For the rest of the observation period through day 14, the study continues safety assessments and collects laboratory and clinical measures of efficacy.

In this study, the planners elect to use a refinement of the CRM approach to increase the quantity of data gathered and perhaps the quality of information as well. The plan calls for increasing cohort size with each succeeding cohort. As the study advances through cohorts, the dose moves closer to the optimal dose that may hold long-term interest. Expanded cohorts thus provide additional data on the most promising doses to aid in planning the remainder of the study and any subsequent studies.

The first cohort consists of one subject on the test drug plus one on placebo. With each cohort, the number of subjects receiving the test drug increases by 1. The number of subjects receiving placebo remains constant at 1. The pattern continues until the study accumulates a comparison pool of a maximum of 10 subjects receiving placebo. Thereafter, the study administers only doses of the test drug. Figure 6-2 shows a schematic representation of this procedure.

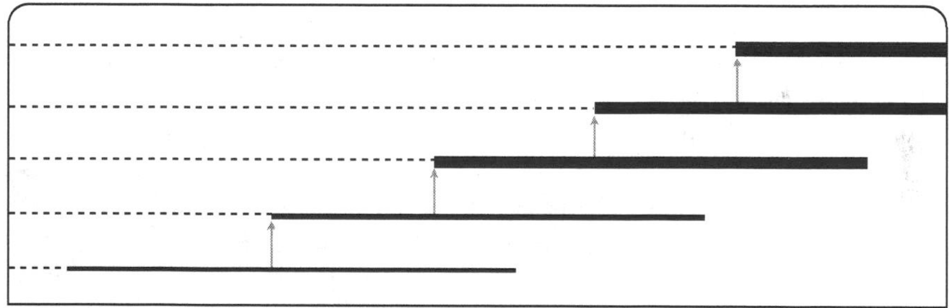

Figure 6-2. Dose-escalation schematic showing succession of cohorts. The vertical lines indicate safety assessment, the basis for determining the dose to be administered the next cohort. The remainder of the horizontal line represents time devoted to observing efficacy as well as ongoing safety. Increasing thickness of horizontal lines represents the growing size of succeeding cohorts. Cohorts increase to gather more data as the dose converges on the optimal.

The initial estimate suggests that there will be little or no treatment effect and no toxicity at a dose of 10 mg. Researchers believe evidence of efficacy is most likely to appear at a dose of 50 mg or greater. They expect to find evidence of toxicity at doses between 100 and 200 mg. Rather than starting at 10 mg and allowing only increments until reaching DLT, the study starts at 50 mg and allows increments or decrements of 25 mg based on patient response.

Planning

A secondary goal for this study, provided all goes well in initial safety and efficacy testing, is to proceed quickly into dose finding. If dose finding also goes as hoped, the goal is to proceed rapidly to confirmatory trials. Provided results warrant, plans allow for seamless transitions between tasks conventionally performed in separate phases with gaps between.

Planners run simulations to examine the effect of different likely dosing levels, lead time for drug supply, and number of sites required. Under different favorable scenarios, simulations also consider approaches to expanding the study population and adding a second confirmatory study to complete the program. Because of the desire to complete the program rapidly, planners decide to utilize two sites for early testing despite the increase in complexity. Two potential benefits more than outweigh the burden of complexity: the ability to recruit and treat cohorts more rapidly and the ability to conduct a low-risk "shakeout" test of systems for later large-scale testing at multiple sites.

Operational Considerations

A primary operational focus is on facilitating rapid decisions on dose increments or decrements. This requires rapid data capture, validation, and analysis. Determination of the dose of each successive cohort considers response data on all previous cohorts. The goal is having the basis for next dosing decisions on day 4, including complete safety data and laboratory evaluations on each cohort. The study follows patients for efficacy data through day 10. However, efficacy information plays no role in determining the next dose. The operational goal is not to wait until the following day to collect and analyze data but to assure the availability of safety results within two hours of final measurement of each cohort. Decisions on dose increments or decrements are to take place within four hours of final measurement. The senior scientists who determine the next dose have agreed to provide continuous review of data generated and to decide whether to increment or decrement the dose within the desired four-hour limit. Since availability of laboratory data is usually the limiting step, the study carefully defines associated procedures, responsibilities, and expectations. Accuracy is imperative. The study uses internal crosschecks to assure rapid validation and correction of any data errors within the two-hour period. Making preliminary results available early facilitates final decisions because the team can consider most of the data before receiving the final pieces. Final results become available immediately upon the recording of the validated outcome for each cohort (Figure 6-2).

To ensure the availability of accurate and reliable data within time constraints, study planners decide to collect data using the digital pen and an associated data-processing system that begins validation on receipt of data. The digital pen allows direct recording of source data. The electronic record is the source data, with a paper image of the data printed if desired. Electronic source data reduces the need for field monitoring by eliminating the need to compare original paper documents with electronic data transcribed from the original. Using the digital pen as source also eliminates transcription and thus the need to recheck transcribed data. The system can provide accurate results within two hours of data collection.

To maximize efficiency by eliminating transfer steps between different systems, the study uses a centralized system that integrates study infrastructure. Integrated functions include randomization, drug-supply tracking, storing and viewing data on drug response, and determining when to suspend enrollment until completion of a cohort and review of its data before the next dosing decision. The integration of randomization and the supply system prevents communication delays that can allow continued randomization of patients to already full cohorts. A flow chart defines proper procedures for all key members of the study team, whether at the test site, at offices for internal staff, or at offices of decision makers. The entire team must agree to observe tight deadlines throughout. An additional operational safeguard is training backup personnel for each key role to prevent an absence from compromising timelines.

Putting the Plan into Action

Recognizing the importance of maintaining tight schedules, study managers create a detailed operational plan for executing the safety study. The plan includes flow charts and timelines. It also designates individuals responsible for key activities at each step. Each member of the study team has a list of individual responsibilities, including tasks, procedures, and timing. Contingency plans identify backup personnel for each activity. Contingency planning considers scenarios such as illness, missing specimens, laboratory difficulties, availability of computer support, and possible interruptions of information flow.

The small group of individuals charged with making dosing decisions pledge their availability on short notice even if traveling. Plans require 75% of decision makers to agree on dose escalations. To accelerate decision making, study managers require a standard, continuously updated report summarizing safety data to date. The report specifies a series of safety measurements and provides a visual summary of the data. Reports of individual assessments appear in a form resembling that shown in Figure 6-3.

After five dosing cycles, the decision group feels the accumulated information justifies the transition to larger-scale testing focused on dose finding. The transition is seamless and provided for continued safety testing during dose finding with larger groups.

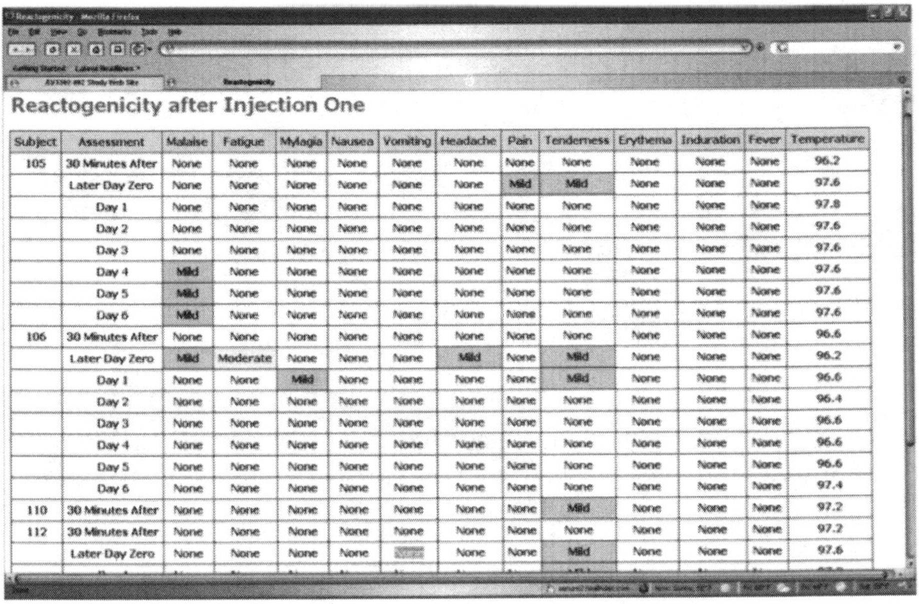

Reactogenicity after Injection One

Subject	Assessment	Malaise	Fatigue	Mylagia	Nausea	Vomiting	Headache	Pain	Tenderness	Erythema	Induration	Fever	Temperature
105	30 Minutes After	None	None	None	None	None	None	None	None	None	None	None	96.2
	Later Day Zero	None	None	None	None	None	None	Mild	Mild	None	None	None	97.6
	Day 1	None	None	None	None	None	None	None	None	None	None	None	97.8
	Day 2	None	None	None	None	None	None	None	None	None	None	None	97.6
	Day 3	None	None	None	None	None	None	None	None	None	None	None	97.6
	Day 4	Mild	None	None	None	None	None	None	None	None	None	None	97.6
	Day 5	Mild	None	None	None	None	None	None	None	None	None	None	97.6
	Day 6	Mild	None	None	None	None	None	None	None	None	None	None	97.6
106	30 Minutes After	None	None	None	None	None	None	None	None	None	None	None	96.6
	Later Day Zero	Mild	Moderate	None	None	None	Mild	None	Mild	None	None	None	96.2
	Day 1	None	None	Mild	None	None	None	None	Mild	None	None	None	96.6
	Day 2	None	None	None	None	None	None	None	None	None	None	None	96.4
	Day 3	None	None	None	None	None	None	None	None	None	None	None	96.6
	Day 4	None	None	None	None	None	None	None	None	None	None	None	96.6
	Day 5	None	None	None	None	None	None	None	None	None	None	None	96.6
	Day 6	None	None	None	None	None	None	None	None	None	None	None	97.4
110	30 Minutes After	None	None	None	None	None	None	None	Mild	None	None	None	97.2
112	30 Minutes After	None	None	None	None	None	None	None	None	None	None	None	97.2
	Later Day Zero	None	None	None	None	[illegible]	None	None	Mild	None	None	None	97.6

Figure 6-3. Summary of safety data for each subject. This data becomes available within two hours of completing the observation period. Determination of the dose for the next cohort takes place within four hours. Additional data displays summarize safety as well as efficacy data.

Source: Health Decisions, Inc. Copyright 2006. Used by permission.

Benefits Realized

Using the CRM approach for safety testing allowed reducing the number and duration of decision cycles. The total time for each dosing decision shrank from the typical 17 days (4 days of observation, 10 days to process and present data, 3 days to make decisions) to only 4 days, a 76% reduction. The net savings for this phase was 2.6 months. Utilizing the CRM dose-finding method and starting a third of the way up the dose-response curve saved two dosing cycles, allowing the study to define safety and efficacy in four cycles. This improved on the six cycles required by a conventional approach and required 33% fewer subjects.

Establishing a pool of subjects treated with placebo produced a small additional savings—in this case, a single subject, resulting in 39% fewer subjects than with a traditional approach. Early testing at two sites rather than the usual one added complexity and increased baseline costs (site contracts, IRBs) at the outset by about 25%. However, program managers expected this shakedown of multisite management procedures to provide benefits in later phases. Modeling possible outcomes took some time but provided a sounder basis for decision making, reducing the likelihood of false steps.

The direct cost savings were substantial, including a 70% reduction in monitoring time compared to a conventional model. These savings came primarily from reducing requirements for source verification through use of electronic source data and remote site management based on continuous quality measures. These same capabilities helped ensure rapid availability of reliable data. Rapid validation also promoted rapid site and study closeout. The need to ensure accurate data to support midcourse decision making enabled the study team to resolve issues early that are often not discovered until a study ends. In sum, the agile approach saved 69% of costs, 76% of time, and 39% in number of subjects as compared to a traditional program (Figure 6-4).

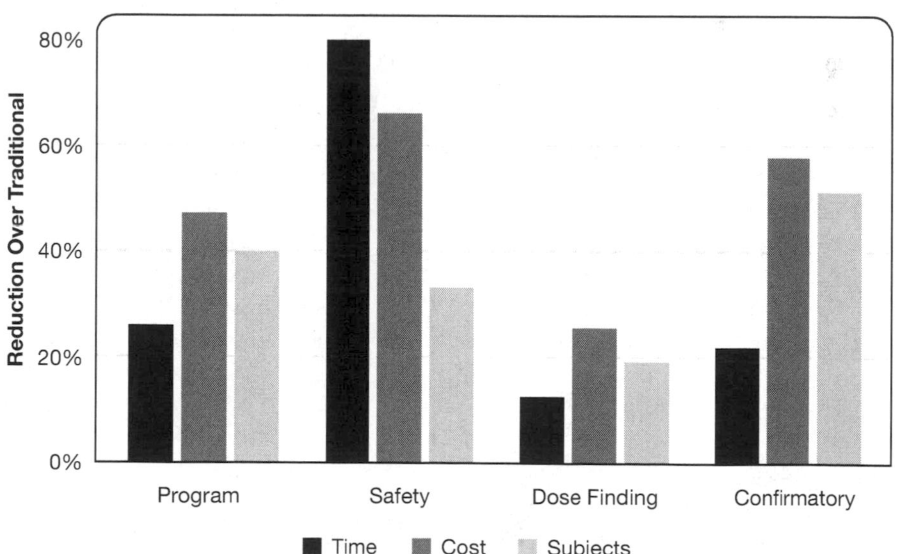

Figure 6-4. Use of the agile approach for safety testing of the hypothetical test drug saved 78 days and $50,000 and exposed seven fewer subjects to the experimental treatment.

Transition to Dose-Finding

Planners designed this study from the outset for a seamless transition from first safety testing into dose finding. Such a design was one reason for attention to efficacy measures in early evaluations. At the beginning of the safety-testing phase, planners outlined the protocol for the following dose-finding phase and defined the timeline for steps needed to minimize the transition. These steps included site identification, protocol refinement, and initial and final IRB submissions.

To save time, sites initiate early contact with IRBs and establish a two-step approval with a first review before the end of safety testing and final review at study completion. The existence of a well-defined regulatory pathway for the indication and drug class helps make this approach possible. Early planning meetings to identify steps and criteria for rapid progression of the development program also help.

Midway through the safety evaluation, study planners begin developing the plan for the following dose-finding study, deciding the number of dosing arms and number and distribution of sites. Based on simulations, planners identify and begin initiating eight sites. Sites and sponsors work closely with IRBs to ensure expedited, two-step IRB review of the final dose-finding protocol. Planners call for completing detailed preparations for the dose-finding phase at the three-quarter point of early safety testing. This includes completing protocol refinements, CRFs, workflow definitions, and arrangements for supplies of the test drug and other materials.

The plan for the transition calls for a gap of no more than two weeks between close of the safety phase and the initiation of the dose-finding efforts. By prearrangement, study managers prepare a summary of results for regulators on completing the safety phase. The sponsor submits this summary within a week of completion. To speed preparation of the report, study managers and statisticians prepare preliminary versions of the report using partial data, then substitute final data. Monitors complete site closeout visits within a week. The study team completes updating reports with final figures over the following week. The team submits the reports in parallel with initiation of the dose-finding phase. In the same period, the study team ensures completion of final IRB changes, expedited by prior approval of preliminary submissions. As planned, the study completed the transition to dose finding within two weeks.

Dose Finding (Phase II)

Design

This phase seeks to establish efficacy (proof of concept), select active arms for confirmatory testing, and establish comparators, both active and placebo. The use of both active and placebo comparators is unusual. Planners power the study to demonstrate a significantly improved efficacy score compared with placebo, with secondary goals of exploring noninferiority or superiority relative to the active comparator. The former strategy seeks to establish early proof of concept. The latter strategy seeks to identify the better claim for use in confirmatory testing. The active comparator is a currently available product using a different route of administration (injection).

The plan also includes sample-size reestimation. There are two interim looks for this purpose, the first when 50% and the second when 75% of the data is in. A separate decision-making group of senior company officials, firewalled from study personnel, also monitors study data continuously.

The dose-finding phase starts with a larger than usual number of arms and prunes arms based on patient response. Regulators agree to allow the sponsor to prune arms flexibly at any point, with the sponsor responsible for assuring safety and efficacy. Study planners must define the standard of safety and efficacy before the study by comparison with the active comparator, based on knowledge about the marketed product. Regulatory authorities also allow sponsors the option of electing to terminate the study early without performing a formal frequentist statistical analysis.

Another objective of the dose-finding phase of this program is to explore the utility of the surrogate marker as an outcome measure. Regulatory authorities have agreed to consider allowing use of this marker as a primary indicator for confirmatory studies, based on data from at least 300 subjects. The sponsor considers this possibility remote because of the regulatory group's traditional reluctance to allow use of surrogates in confirmatory studies.

The design calls for a seamless transition from dose finding into confirmatory testing. To enable the rapid transition, study planners must conduct the dose-finding phase precisely as though it were a confirmatory study from the outset. This requires additional internal protections to ensure that individuals tasked with assessing the interim results are independent of those conducting the study. In this hypothetical program, the sponsor simplifies implementation of this approach by using a CRO with experience conducting adaptive studies and managing associated logistical issues.

Planning

The study is to begin with six active and two comparator arms. Planners establish criteria for efficacy based on existing regulatory guidance for this class of drug and the indication treated. Sample-size reestimation relies on a conventional frequentist approach that includes a prespecified low alpha spend for both scheduled interim looks. The study plan calls for two independent review groups, the first an external data-monitoring committee focused on protecting participant interests. The second review group consists of senior officials from the sponsoring company. This second group will make decisions about terminating dosing arms or the entire study. The mission of this second group is to assess the project in light of the company's competing projects and business environment.

Simulation determines initial sample size based on the most conservative estimates of a superiority indication against the active comparator. Because history indicates a higher and earlier dropout for placebo subjects, this simulation includes differential dropout rates for placebo groups and all active arms. Simulation estimates a 90% probability of a maximum of 480 subjects, 50% probability of 390, and 10% probability of 280. However, the potential for variation is great, depending on how many arms the study terminates and when. After using simulation to explore a range of possibilities, planners decide to go with 75% of the 90% probability figure, or 75 subjects in each arm and 360 altogether. This approach is conservative; earlier cutoffs would allow using fewer subjects.

Planners deliberate the number of sites required. During safety evaluations, study planners rank 15 qualified sites according to three main criteria: enrollment capability, responsiveness, and ability to work with project and data management systems, the last assessed based on considerations such as the quality of site coordinators. Planners narrow the list to 6 sites for initiation. However, planners also divide the remaining sites into two backup groups. The study team informs all sites to expect exclusion from the study if they fail to enroll a patient within two months. When expanding for confirmatory testing, the study will include all sites that meet expectations in the dose-finding phase.

The analysis considers the number of sites, different levels of enrollment performance, and their effect on study duration (Figure 6-5). With sites estimating an average enrollment of eight subjects per month, study managers decide to use 6 sites. This assumes discontinuation of 2 sites for poor enrollment.

Recognizing the importance of drug supply, the planners recommend using a system that integrates drug supply with data input and site information. With the centralized system, records of randomization and visits appropriately decrement the supplies on hand. Some sites responsible for optional

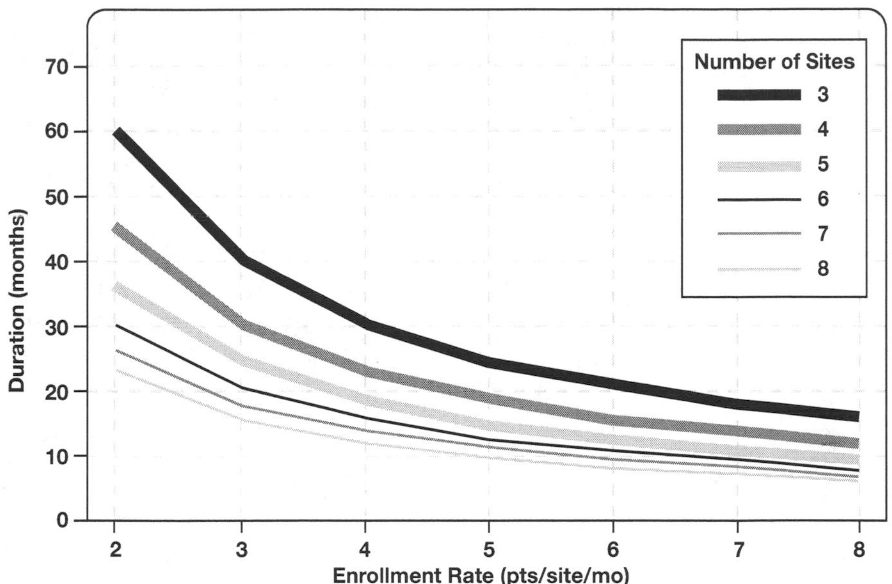

Figure 6-5. Projected duration of the dose-finding study assuming different enrollment rates (horizontal axis) and numbers of sites (tinted lines). Weighing the added complexity of including additional sites against longer study duration with fewer sites, planners decide to include eight sites and cut off nonperformers after two months if necessary, leaving a minimum of six and maximum of eight sites.

clinical evaluations are to receive payment after submitting data on evaluations of their subjects. To encourage sites to minimize and quickly resolve queries, plans call for a monthly contest for fastest response times. The study automates site payments, paying a portion on data submission and the balance on resolution of associated queries for each submission.

Finally, planners look ahead to the hoped-for confirmatory studies to follow dose finding. Early on, planners recognize the need to include European sites, in part because other studies are targeting the same patient population in the United States.

Operational Considerations

The study uses adaptive monitoring, with dynamic assignment of monitors. Monitoring visits occur at intervals averaging eight weeks. The first monitoring visit takes place early, preferably around the time of the first patient visit. The frequency of additional monitoring visits depends on prespecified site performance metrics. The frequency of visits increases or decreases based on number of patients enrolled and quality and quantity of data submitted. Study managers plan monitoring visits based on availability of an appropriate amount of data for review within the timeframe specified for each visit. Availability of detailed metrics on the rate at which each field monitor can perform tasks allows matching monitoring schedules with individual capabilities.

Recognizing the need to align the interests of sites with those of the sponsor to ensure completing the study quickly, the study uses key site performance indicators including rates for screen failure, enrollment, discontinuation, queries, and query response times. Comparative data for all sites provides a level of detail that allows managers to determine where improvements are possible at each site. Sites meeting prespecified criteria in each area qualify for participation in the confirmatory study; other sites do not. A dedicated study website tracks a competitive enrollment process and displays comparative performance for all sites.

Knowing that the scarcity of patients and existence of competing studies will complicate enrollment, the study team formulates enrollment strategies with care. At the outset, the study will use several approaches. The study will closely track the pace of enrollment using each strategy. Contingency plans include expansion of advertising efforts as well as adding additional sites. Sites can determine their own recruitment strategies based on knowledge of local patient populations, referral patterns, media, and other factors. However, study management provides a choice of three recruitment messages for posting in site waiting rooms and three different messages for posting on internet forums where patients discuss experiences with the health condition. The study also tests a radio spot ad for two sites and a newspaper ad for two others.

Putting the Plan into Action

The study quickly initiates sites, with three-quarters starting patient enrollment during the first month. One more site joins the second month and another the third. However, study managers drop one site for failure to enroll the prescribed number of patients. This leaves the study with seven enrolling sites.

Patient recruitment remains a high priority because it affects the ability to meet timelines. The study tracks patient referrals closely, assessing the performance of sources and messages. The effort soon establishes that waiting room notices and internet postings are most effective, with both directing patients toward telephone screeners who refer qualified patients to a local site. The study shifts resources to focus on using the successful recruitment message for all sites. Enrollment accelerates. The study ends the less cost-effective radio spots and newspaper ads. However, the study decides to maintain efforts at several internet forums with slight changes in the messaging.

Within 24 hours of data submission, the study management system returns automated queries. Close tracking of data detects patterns that identify several operational issues:

- There are high query rates across all sites on two CRF fields. Central monitoring based on automated performance metrics and rapid analysis suggests the problem is overly restrictive validation rules: one on blood pressure, which specifies a narrow acceptable range of 80–120 for systolic, the other on poor wording of the question. The study manager authorizes resetting validation limits. The study team analyzes CRF instructions, improves wording, and communicates the new instructions immediately to all sites through the study website and e-mails. Monitoring visits also call attention to these changes. Query rates on these CRF questions fall dramatically.
- The query rate for one site more than doubles in a short period. Closer examination of data and comparison of this site with study averages show queries spiking not for one or two fields but for many. A call to the site quickly identifies the problem: a personnel change unknown to the CRO. Having missed training, the new staff member at the site is deviating from instructions for one procedure and completing CRFs incorrectly as well. The study team immediately initiates online training modules, interactive webcast, and calls from monitors to ensure understanding of study requirements and procedures. A possible extra visit for training proves unnecessary. However, the site's monitor focuses on this issue at the next visit. The query rate quickly drops into the range expected for a new employee. The monitor continues to track that employee's performance.
- A month into the study, data shows that about 20% of screen failures are for a hemoglobin level of less than 10 grams. Many patients fail for values slightly below the minimum. After internal staff consults clinicians with relevant expertise, the study seeks regulatory approval to reduce the minimum acceptable level to 9.5 grams. Regulators grant the request. Study managers implement a protocol amendment and obtain expedited IRB approval. Screen failures drop 10%. Other minor changes to inclusion and exclusion criteria allow enrollment to increase 15% within three months.

Centralized study personnel also work closely with sites to help analyze workflow, identify chokepoints, smooth operations, and reduce rework. Quick responses on queries result in a rapid reduction in query rates to slightly less than one query per 100 fields (<1%). All sites meet requested response times, and competitive performance metrics result in steady improvement. Centralized managers also work closely with slow-enrolling sites, tracking site-specific recruitment rates against overall study rates. Managers identify projected monthly goals to allow the sites to meet commitments. Comparative metrics help focus the sites on recruitment. Centralized study managers intervene quickly when necessary, working with the site coordinator. The managers train other site personnel to assist with CRF completion and query resolution while the coordinator focuses on enrollment. Enrollment accelerates.

The overall enrollment rate per site increases slightly with time, eventually settling at 7 patients per site per month. However, the number of patients enrolled in each active arm increases from an average of 7.2 during the first month of enrollment to 12.3 in the final, a 24% improvement.

Study managers adjust design in several respects:

- Discontinuing the placebo arm. Continuous tracking of early results shows response in all treated groups clearly superior to placebo. The placebo group also experiences a substantially higher dropout rate than treated groups. The internal oversight group terminates the placebo arm for ethical reasons.
- Reestimating sample size. Midway through the study, the treatment effect is lower than original estimates, and the dropout rate in the placebo group exceeds estimates but is lower than estimated in high-dose treatment groups. The net result is a 9% reduction in total sample size, to 68 patients per group.
- Reducing the "insurance buffer" on sample size. Given the measured effects and consistency over time, study managers reduce the buffer from 20% to 10%.
- Initiating confirmatory studies as planned for favorable scenarios. Because results look positive, study managers begin identification and initiation of additional sites for confirmatory studies in month 6 and conduct discussions with European regulators.
- A second sample-size reestimation at the three-quarter mark. Data indicates values from the previous reestimation are holding. The sponsor elects to retain the 10% "insurance" margin. The study implements plans for expansion and transition into the confirmatory phase, including submission of previously-agreed-upon regulatory reports to allow direct transition to confirmatory testing.
- Dropping the lowest-performing active arm, based on data at the three-quarter mark.

Following careful planning and progressive lock by visit and subject, the study team locks the database three days after LPLV. Two weeks of intensive analysis allow completion of the study report for submission to regulatory officials.

Benefits Realized

Had the sponsor chosen to proceed conventionally, the study would have taken 22 months (14 months to recruit, another 8 to complete patient visits and follow-up), required 446 patients, and cost, at an average of $20,000 per patient, $8.5 million. The agile approach incorporating design adaptations and operational refinements allowed completing the study in 10.5 months with 360 patients, per-patient cost of $17,500, and total cost of $6.3 million. Figure 6-6 compares the traditional and agile approaches to dose finding on the hypothetical scenario described. The agile approach provided savings of 11.5 months (52%), 86 patients (19%), and $2.2 million (26%). Because the agile approach allowed completing enrollment, treatment, and follow-up faster, the agile study incurred patient costs faster, too. The traditional study would spread its higher patient costs over a much longer period because of slower execution.

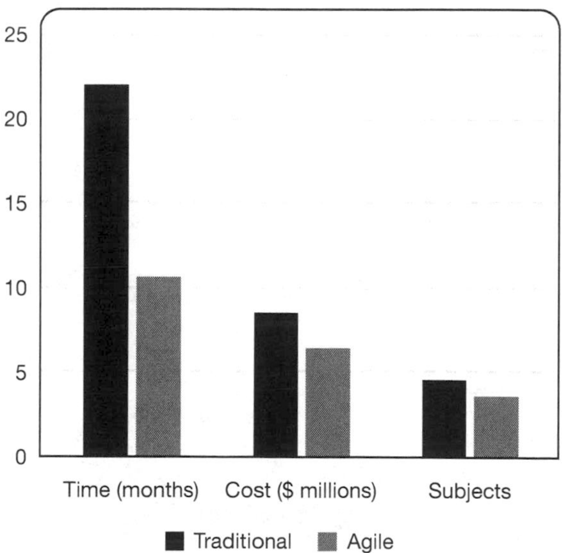

Figure 6-6. On the hypothetical scenario described, agile methods for dose finding saved 11.5 months and $2.2 million and required exposing 86 fewer patients to the experimental treatment.

Transition to Confirmatory Studies

A two-step review by prearrangement with regulators allows a rapid transition to confirmatory testing. The study continues to observe patients enrolled in the arms carried over from the dose-finding portion of the trial while enrolling new patients to increase study size for confirmatory requirements. Since the study data meets preapproved criteria, the sponsor moves aggressively during the two-month review to prepare the launch of the confirmatory phase.

An important consideration at this point is possible use of the surrogate measure. This measure correlates reasonably well with both the three-month outcome and the six-month observation period for patients enrolled before month 6. Unresolved regulatory questions include whether the surrogate measure could serve in lieu of established longer-term outcomes or as an early indicator allowing initiation of marketing plans while awaiting longer-term outcomes. The study submits data to regulatory authorities. The data meets previously agreed-upon performance measures, including assessment of the surrogate measure. However, not having received regulatory approval for use of the surrogate, the sponsor proceeds on the assumption that the surrogate is unacceptable.

Confirmatory Testing (Phase III)

Design

By prior agreement with regulators, the sponsor is rolling the dose-finding portion of the seamless trial into a confirmatory study that will generate frequentist statistics appropriate for a regulatory submission. The observation period for confirmatory testing will be longer than for previous phases. The seamless design will allow carrying data forward on patients in arms that continue into the confirmatory phase.

Both sample size and geographic scope will expand. The study will identify and initiate both U.S. and European sites. Simulations again help set sample size, establishing a goal of 120 patients per arm. An important determinant of the sample size is the estimated dropout rate during extended observation periods. The sample-size estimate adjusts for anticipated dropouts and patients lost to follow-up.

Plans call for sample-size reestimation after collection of half the expected data in the first confirmatory study, which has shortened timelines because the analysis includes the 68 patients in the dose 3 and dose 4 and one comparison group. The data review for sample-size reestimation fine-tunes enrollment objectives. It also seeks to establish a clear enough distinction between dosing arms to allow discontinuing the worst-performing arm. The plan calls for minimizing the alpha spend at this point. The decision to drop an arm will not rely on formal hypothesis testing.

Planning

Plans called for identification of additional sites starting when data from the dose-finding phase indicated that the drug was effective and the sponsor judged that the drug would have a promising market niche. A first confirmatory study will expand the dose-finding study already underway, but the sponsor will also schedule a second confirmatory study using the same protocol to accelerate regulatory submissions.

Study planners address a variety of enrollment contingencies. Given the larger sample size and the belief that U.S. sites are close to saturation, study managers identify 25 additional sites. Of these, study managers believe 10 will be adequate for study needs based on a more modest enrollment rate of six patients per site per month, as observed in the dose-finding portion. Contingency plans provide for keeping five additional sites in different degrees of readiness and activating as necessary. The number activated will depend on enrollment rates at existing sites. Because of a competing trial in the United States, most contingency sites are European. Using European sites will add complexity because of the need for regulatory submissions as a starting point. The sponsor is to complete regulatory submissions as rapidly as possible for countries where the first of four contingency sites are located. Each site is to make arrangements with IRB and local review committees that allow bringing sites online in an estimated two-month window. Upon initiation of the first tier of sites, the same process is to begin at the second tier of contingency sites.

Simulation again aids in determining initial sample size for the second confirmatory study based on data from the dose-finding effort. Because the data is recent and the plan for the study includes sample-size reestimation, planners decide a 5% buffer would provide adequate "insurance" for the study. Planners power the study to have a 95% probability of showing an effect at least as great as the smallest difference present in the previous dose-finding effort. Planners determine a sample size of 120 completers per arm based on simulation involving main determinants such as enrollment rate and dropout rate.

The confirmatory studies are to focus from the outset on measures to facilitate rapid site closeout and database lock. The planning steps required involve defining all queries to be resolved in the final weeks of the study and specifying all requirements for last-day activities. These tasks are to start with measurement of all outstanding queries, number of queries expected during remaining data collection efforts for the study, monitoring efforts required to complete source verification, and coordination with labs to analyze and provide results quickly.

The second confirmatory study is to launch simultaneously with expansion of the first confirmatory study, reflecting a commitment to early regulatory filing.

Operational

Operational plans include a range of strategies for improving efficiency:

- The digital pen will serve as the primary means of data collection, including for patient diaries. However, study managers decide two sites with poor communications and a need for greater oversight should use paper optical mark recording CRFs. Sites record about 30% of data directly on digital pen CRFs as source, obviating the need for source data verification on this information. Some sites that would normally record study data in other records use the digital pen as source with provision for immediately returning a report by e-mail to the site in a form suitable for printing and pasting into patient charts.
- The study will use a combination of local monitoring and close centralized management.
- Recognizing the importance of minimizing patients lost to follow-up, study managers establish a procedure for quick intervention when patients miss appointments to ensure rapid follow-up by sites. Follow-up is to include determining the reasons for missing appointments and increasingly intense efforts to retain patients, including, if necessary, paying for extraordinary transportation and having site personnel visit patients.
- The confirmatory studies will use adaptive monitoring, with intervals between site visits adjusted throughout the study according to quality and quantity of data submitted by each site. Intervals average 10 weeks.
- Study managers use incremental closeout throughout the study. To facilitate quick study closure, study managers prepare detailed lists of closeout visits and plan for additional monitors to avoid delays if numerous patients complete the study simultaneously.

Putting the Plan into Action

- Enrollment at first averages only four patients per site per month. Enrollment tracking for the first two months shows wide variation in referral rates and screen-failure rates at different sites. The enrollment strategies that worked in previous efforts in the U.S. do not work as well in Europe. However, European sites get good results by emphasizing physician referrals. One country gets best results by using more frequent reminders and additional, locally developed recruitment materials. Sites in another country rely on identifying patients through health service registries and sending individual letters to primary physicians. Shared experience leads investigators to focus on two primary strategies that increase overall enrollment to an average of 8 patients per site per month across the study.
- The first confirmatory study carries forward 86 patients treated during the dose-finding study. Enrollment for the first confirmatory study reaches the halfway point after two additional months, and data is available on 94 patients in each of three groups (dose 4, dose 3, comparator).
- Sample-size reestimation halfway through the planned recruitment period reveals a higher-than-expected response rate in the comparison arm. This requires increasing sample size 9%, to 130 patients per arm, to retain desired power.
- Sample-size reestimation reveals an unexpectedly high response rate in the placebo group. This also reveals little difference between clinical efficacy measures of the two doses but a modestly increased safety concern with the higher dose. Study managers decide to drop the arm with the higher dose in both confirmatory studies and increase enrollment rates in both studies to an average of 32 patients per month.
- Patient retention exceeds estimates. Study managers attribute this to close tracking that allows quick identification of patients who fail to return as scheduled or may be at high risk of dropping out, as well as intensive follow-up with both. Although better retention rates could allow enrolling fewer patients, study managers take into account the limited information available at the time of SSRE, especially about long-term trends, and make the conservative decision not to decrease enrollment targets.
- Better-than-planned patient retention rates hold for the remainder of the study, with final figures about 14% better than planning estimates.

- After interim review, encouraging results justify starting preparation of regulatory submission in earnest. To this end, detailed planning begins for rapid database lock. Key actions include emphasis on eliminating problems that lead to needless queries; encouraging rapid query resolution through incentives, disincentives, and other measures; and ensuring that a monitor is on site for the last patient's last visit.

Adaptive monitoring increases efficiency greatly. Study managers use adaptive monitoring techniques to address several issues. For example:

- Close adaptive monitoring tracks underperforming sites to identify reasons for poor performance. The most common reason is failure by sites to communicate clear expectations, supervise personnel closely, or help personnel address problems. The central managers step in to help site personnel prioritize work. Some earlier-than-planned monitoring trips allow managers to work directly with site personnel.
- Several sites fail to improve despite repeated efforts at helping identify and manage problems. These sites persistently underperform in basic measures such as time for CRF submission and query resolution. Centralized study managers ask sites to assign replacement staff and follow up with a site visit allowing the monitor to review study procedures and expectations and stress the desire for a team approach. These measures rapidly improve site performance.
- Close tracking of incoming data allows the central monitoring team to notice within a week of patient visits when several patients at one site experience unexpected departures from a trend of relatively stable disease state. The monitoring manager discovers that the trained administrator has been out sick, leaving an untrained secretary to administer assessments. The study team initiates training immediately, delaying scheduled assessments until training is complete.
- Central managers help site personnel focus efforts on the study's priorities. When some sites fall behind in query resolution, central managers help focus sites on first resolving open queries related to subjects who have discontinued or completed the study.
- Central managers closely track missed patient visits. When a site fails to submit expected data on a visit, central personnel call to determine whether the visit occurred. Missed visits not yet rescheduled trigger actions to locate the patient, a task that busy site personnel might have missed or put off.
- Central managers orchestrate discussions among sites for peer-to-peer information sharing. In one instance, managers organize a small

weekend conference for sites that had consistently underperformed, resulting in rapid improvement.

- Progressive closeout throughout the study closes each subject as soon as possible, minimizing work left until the end.

These adaptive monitoring efforts deliver impressive results:

- Adaptive monitoring reduces costs by $4,000 per patient, a 17% reduction in per-patient costs. A low query rate of 0.9/100 fields shows the efficiency of adaptive monitoring.
- Adaptive monitoring allows rapid site closeout and database lock. At the time of the last patient visit, sites submit data and the study team completes validation an hour and a half after the last patient leaves a site. This includes returning queries, revalidating, returning additional queries, and resolving the last query or queries.

To complete the process of rapid database lock, study managers arrange for lab results to come in one day following LPLV. Initial database lock takes place the day after LPLV. Resolution of existing serious adverse events, coding, and internal review requires an additional week.

The statistics group issues top-line results the same evening. Success! Results for the drug closely match predictions from the last analysis. The follow-up rate observed at the interim review holds, and final levels exceed original estimates for patient retention. The study concludes with slightly more patients than needed for the specified statistical power.

Benefits Realized

By including the 68 patients from the dose-finding effort and eliminating the dose 3 arm, the first study met the enrollment target of 130 patients early in month 4. However, the second confirmatory began enrollment at month 0 and completed enrollment halfway through month 6, with an average enrollment of 20 patients per month for all eight active sites. This difference allowed extra time to close the first study and plan timely closeout of the second. The last patient's last visit for the first confirmatory study occurred in month 10. The second study reached the same milestone 2 months afterward. Careful preparation and early query resolution helped reduce time to database lock to only 1 month. Thus, the study completed both confirmatory studies in 13 months. Although circumstances for the two studies differed somewhat, they used the same fundamental plan and protocols and produced similar results.

Conducting the two confirmatory studies with traditional methods would have taken 38 months, with 18 months to enroll, 17 months to complete treatment and follow-up, and 3 months to lock the database and analyze. The traditional confirmatory studies would have involved 784 patients and cost, at an average of $23,000 per patient, $18.0 million. The agile approach to both design and operations allowed conducting two confirmatory studies that acquired the same information in 13 months, with 6 months to enroll, 6 months for treatment and follow-up, and 1 month for database lock. The two agile confirmatory studies would have required 705 patients and, at an average of $20,000 per patient, would have cost $14.1 million. Adaptive monitoring reduced per-patient costs with the agile approach. Costs include contingency plans for additional sites, some activated, others not. Figure 6-7 compares the results of the traditional and agile approaches to conducting the two confirmatory studies. These reductions represent savings for the confirmatory studies of 66% in time, 22% in costs, and 10% in number of patients. By far the greatest benefit of the agile approach in these studies is reducing development time and thus accelerating regulatory filing and market entry.

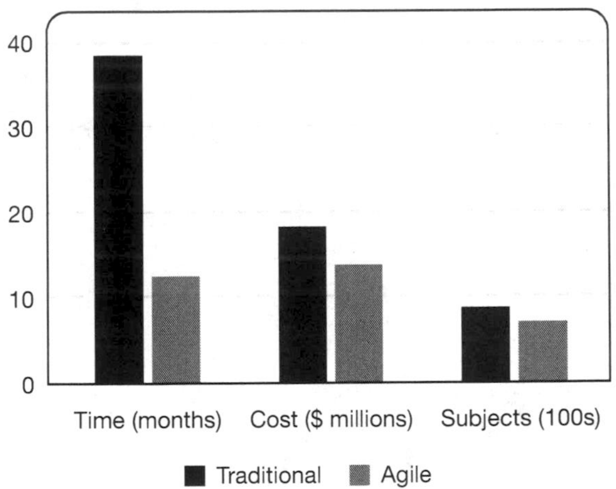

Figure 6-7. Comparison summarizing time, cost, and patient requirements for conducting two confirmatory studies with the traditional approach and equivalent studies with the agile approach.

A conventional version of the confirmatory studies might have faced even more serious problems than higher costs and longer timelines. The different-from-expected response rate in one group, observed at the time of interim analysis, could have prevented demonstrating a difference between the test drug and a comparator. The confirmatory studies might have failed.

Transition to Regulatory Filings

Because of quicker site closeout and database lock and starting work on regulatory submissions seven months before completion of the study, the agile confirmatory studies completed regulatory filings for both Europe and the United States two months faster than is usual for traditional confirmatory studies. Early work on regulatory filing included summaries, draft text, tables, listings, and the shell of a clinical study report, all updated as final data became available. Management activities to support these tasks included implementing a document management system specialized for regulatory filings, hiring specialized personnel, and other measures to allow rapid regulatory submissions.

Summing Up: The Power of Agile Development

Speed is among the most important benefits of the hypothetical development program, reducing the time required to take the new drug from safety testing to regulatory filing. Figure 6-8 shows how markedly the agile approach could reduce development timelines in this hypothetical case. Savings are substantial, both within phases of development and between phases. The overall reduction is from 7 years, 4 months to 4 years, 4½ months.

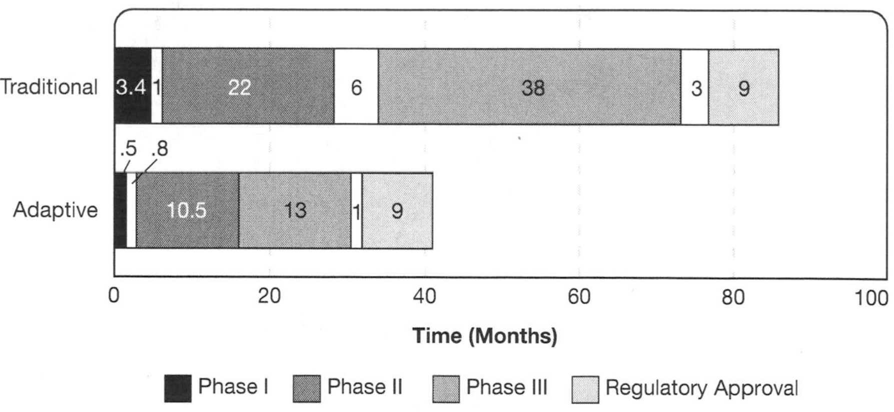

Figure 6-8. By combining a variety of operational adaptations with design adaptations and seamless designs, the agile approach shortens the hypothetical drug development program by more than 50%, in this case from a typical 82.4 months to 34.8 months. The biggest savings were in the time required for dose-finding and confirmatory studies. This example shows results based on assumptions for this specific example; the time savings in any program depend on individual study circumstances and characteristics.

The flexibility of this hypothetical development program would provide impressive savings in time, costs, and patient exposure to an experimental treatment: 47.6 months, $6.2 million, and 172 fewer subjects compared to a conventional program. Figure 6-9 illustrates the estimated savings for the entire development program as well as for each phase of development. Relative time savings would be greatest in early testing. The greatest savings in cost and patient exposure would come in later tests with larger populations. On the scenarios described, the confirmatory studies alone would save $3.9 million.

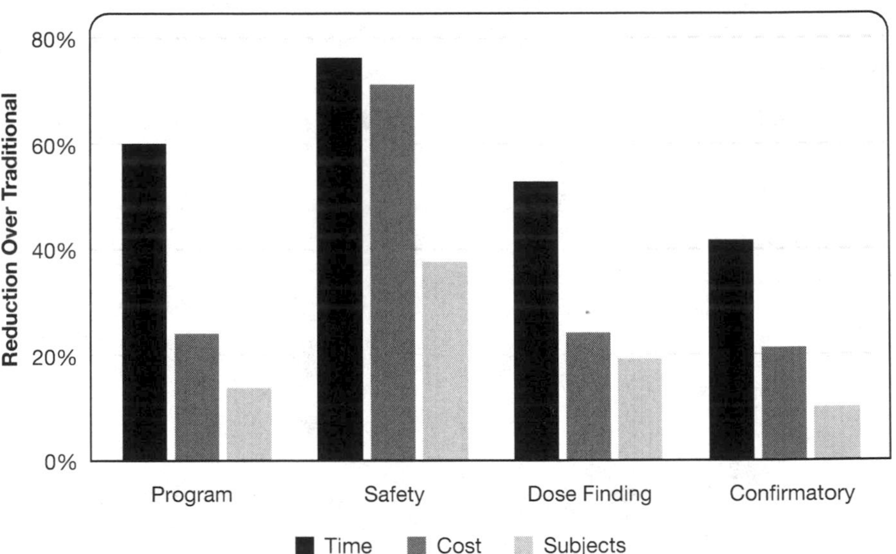

Figure 6-9. Percent savings in time, costs, and number of test subjects that an agile development program provides over a traditional program. Savings are also broken down by development phase.

Although time savings from the agile approach can be substantial, they may not always be the most important benefit. Sometimes earlier acquisition of knowledge matters more. Acquiring greater knowledge earlier allows better-informed decisions about the course of development. The additional knowledge may allow development managers and corporate strategists to create plans that increase prospects of ultimate success. A more nuanced understanding of the test drug in the dose likely to reach market increases the likelihood of successful, long-term use in appropriate patients. Performing better in the marketplace may prove even more valuable than early market entry.

No single scenario can represent a "typical" development program. The scenario described in this chapter is not appropriate for all programs, nor is such a comprehensive application of agile principles an appropriate starting point for adopting the agile approach. Nevertheless, the agile program described here shows a more continuous, flexible approach to clinical development.

Because a conventional program is linear and limited to testing one hypothesis or aspect of a novel drug at a time, choices narrow as the program proceeds. Once testing begins, study and program managers can seldom seize unforeseen opportunities or mitigate the effects of regrettable planning assumptions and strategic choices. By contrast, the flexibility of the agile approach allows a development program to respond to changing circumstances. With careful planning, the agile approach makes it possible to pursue ambitious goals with the security of fallback strategies that offer the prospect of modest success rather than total failure.

Greater freedom to shift emphasis during development is liberating by comparison with traditional linear, all-or-nothing programs. The agile approach increases the range of strategic options at the outset and preserves a greater range of options later in development. In effect, the program can have strategic arms just as a dose-finding study has dosing arms. As the program accumulates information, strategic priorities can change accordingly. Managers can prune fruitless strategies just as dose-finding studies prune futile arms. Effort and resources increasingly focus on the optimal path forward.

The greater strategic freedom and potentially greater rewards of the agile approach come at a price well worth paying. The agile approach requires planning individual studies and entire development programs more thoughtfully. Chapter 7, "Planning Agile Programs," describes the planning challenges and tools for mastering them.

— Chapter 7 —

Planning Adaptive Programs

Planning adaptive programs requires thinking for the long term and devoting even greater than usual attention to detail. Because adaptive programs allow more decision making, planners must consider the long-term consequences of each potential decision. Understanding these consequences requires anticipating an assortment of scenarios. Planning must provide a response for each contingency. Furthermore, planners must ensure the availability of timely, accurate information both to support midcourse decisions and to assess progress toward objectives. Minor oversights can slow a fast-paced program to a crawl. Unanticipated events can halt a program altogether. Although such delays are rare, the mere possibility should motivate the most meticulous possible planning.

Planning of design adaptations is only half the job of planning adaptive studies. Study operations, which provide the vital underpinning for design adaptations, demand similar attention. Decision makers need timely accurate information to determine whether and how to carry out design adaptations. Study managers also need timely accurate information to identify and correct operational problems. The absence of such an adaptive capacity for operations jeopardizes the ability to provide information essential for adapting study designs in midcourse.

Failure to recognize the importance of operational adaptations can make study operations a rate-limiting step for an entire program. Adaptive dose finding and response-adaptive randomization provide examples. Assuming rapid outcomes, each dosing decision depends on how quickly the study can obtain accurate information on the response of test subjects to the latest dose. The ability to follow rules for randomizing subjects also depends on the rapid availability of accurate response information. The choice of dose and randomization ratios may change with each response recorded. Similarly, reducing or eliminating between-study pauses with seamless designs requires the ability to complete essential activities rapidly. This includes resolving queries, closing out sites, locking databases, coordinating with external groups such as IRBs and regulators, and performing many other functions essential for moving to the next phase of testing. All these activities require efficient operations that clean and validate data and identify and resolve problems rapidly.

Planning adaptive programs revolves around setting goals, determining how to measure progress toward goals, and determining how to obtain data required for such measurements. Such planning also requires the ability to forecast likely scenarios and plan appropriate responses for different circumstances at decision points on each scenario.

Determining Design Adaptations and Their Requirements

Planners must specify most aspects of design adaptations in advance. At a minimum, plans for studies involving design adaptations must address:

- aspects of the study design that can change;
- when changes will be considered;
- details of changes allowed (increase, decrease, terminate early, extend, etc.);
- criteria that will determine whether a change is made and in what measure;
- data required to determine whether these criteria are met;
- when decision makers need the data;
- who will decide about changes;
- who will communicate any such decision, how, and to whom;
- how data will be analyzed, by whom, and with what statistical techniques;
- steps necessary to ensure that the analysis takes place within time constraints;
- identification of needs for blinding and policies for defining and maintaining firewalls for protecting internal knowledge;
- implications of adaptations for study logistics and supplies.

Determining Operational Requirements to Support Design Adaptations

Equally important, planners must consider how study operations will ensure the ability to execute design adaptations. Planners must address:

- how to capture the requisite data within time and quality constraints;
- how to ensure timely data validation and query resolution, especially on elements critical for design changes;
- how to ensure that blinding is maintained, if relevant;
- how to ensure the availability of any special capabilities involved, such as real-time randomization;
- how to communicate decisions about design adaptations in a timely manner;
- how to limit access to information involved in making decisions about design adaptations;
- how to determine supply needs.

Ensuring the Ability to Meet Operational Requirements

Study managers must also consider a third category to provide a solid study foundation: how they ensure that study operations attain and maintain the high level of operational efficiency required. Managing operations to such a high level requires addressing:

- establishing performance standards;
- detecting deviations from standards, both negative and positive;
- ensuring the ability to detect operational problems rapidly;
- ensuring the ability to identify and correct problems with underperforming sites;
- improving across all sites any aspects of operations that are amenable to improvement, whether identified as problems or not.

Development managers should never allow operations to falter because of the inability to measure performance, identify problems, and find solutions. Neither should they allow design adaptations to falter because operations fail to provide timely data needed for decision making.

The Importance of Programmatic Thinking

With the agile approach to clinical development, program planning ceases to be about a sequence of separate studies. Planning must envision an integrated, continuous development process as rich in possibilities as that described in Chapter 6. So many possibilities exist that the challenge is planning a program that can efficiently select the optimal path. This includes establishing safety and identifying the most promising dose for testing against the most promising hypothesis. Conventional planning with the primary emphasis on the details of the individual study can no longer cope with the range of possibilities that new techniques and operational improvements have opened up. The number of decisions required to find the optimal path for an entire development program overwhelms familiar planning methods.

Looking Ahead

Adaptive studies potentially allow a look-ahead capability that offers the opportunity to eliminate many conventional bottlenecks and to reduce the time between studies. The best example is a program in which midstudy results can provide a basis for initiating plans for regulatory submissions and subsequent studies. Interim results of a study in progress may help shape not only the course of the study itself but also the evolution of an entire development program. The planning process must also consider important logistical contingencies involved in such possibilities as expanding a study based on initial success, extending the study under different circumstances (such as dropping subpopulations), or suspending or halting development. Interim data can allow earlier and deeper analysis of such possibilities, with analysis refined as data becomes complete.

Advisory and Oversight Groups

Both internal and external review groups play important roles in clinical research, and adaptive research is changing the roles of both. Internal review groups representing the sponsor may be responsible for ensuring the appropriate execution of study procedures. Studies have traditionally charged external groups with responsibility for monitoring patient safety, but outside oversight increasingly includes efficacy as well. The shift from specific safety titles (data safety-monitoring board) to more broad terms (independent data-monitoring committee, IDMC) reflects this change. While the primary task of external groups is to protect patient interests by ensuring impartial review, these external groups play a growing role in adaptive studies, often by reviewing data and criteria for potential changes of design elements. A balance exists, however, between the function of patient advocate and more substantive involvement in program development, and it is easy to blur the distinction, often to the detriment of the sponsor.

Adaptive trials must clearly delineate the responsibilities and timelines of external committees. Study planning must give each such group an unambiguous mandate and a detailed written description of responsibilities and expectations. Preferably, the study protocol will include these elements. It is particularly important to distinguish between the power to recommend and the power to decide. Can a committee charged with analysis stop a study under certain conditions (say, if a futility boundary is crossed), or does ultimate authority rest with another group or the sponsor? If study data crosses an inferiority boundary, does the committee have the power to drop part of the population and adjust hypotheses?

With the increased flexibility of adaptive trials, decision making must often consider the business implications of midcourse developments. For example, if a drug in development shows lesser efficacy than expected, there must be a decision as to whether to continue development on the same track, reduce the project's priority, or terminate the program. Such a decision has inescapable implications that extend beyond statistics and medicine. It seems unreasonable to expect sponsors with investments at risk to cede such important development decisions, especially to a group with experience and expertise in statistical analysis of safety issues. If an IDMC has broad responsibilities that include making strategic business decisions, planners must consider selecting committee members based on their ability to make such decisions wisely.

More likely, efficacy assessments should trigger recommendations from independent committees. Later-stage trials often have unambiguous criteria that trigger specific actions. For example, crossing a predefined futility boundary would normally result in abandoning the trial. However, sometimes things change within the trial or the world changes around it. Internal information such as relative response of subpopulations or external information from other studies of the test drug or competitive drugs may modify the playing field in unanticipated ways. Therefore, it seems most reasonable to expect final decisions to rest with sponsors. Independent groups privy to unblinded data can contribute invaluable input.

A large issue is separating groups charged with development decisions from those running the study, preventing transmission of any knowledge of results to those actually performing the study. While no firewall can be foolproof, computer access controls and precisely defined work processes can greatly decrease the risk of unauthorized access to information. Simple precautions include convening a review group at a separate location and providing analytic tools and data storage on separate systems, perhaps involving outside service providers.

Optimizing the Planning Process

One pharma executive recently confided, "I know the [adaptive] systems you are talking about can shorten clinical timelines, but my problem is slow internal decision making." The implication is that the time lost in decision making dwarfs the possible gains from more efficient study designs and research methods. Prolonged deliberations at high levels probably reflect admirable determination to write the perfect plan and obtain universal sign-off. However, program management should never allow the time devoted to well-intentioned planning reviews to cancel out the intended benefits of the plans. The clock on a clinical trial should start to tick not with site selection or enrollment of the first patient but with the submission of an internal proposal to conduct a trial. Improving the efficiency of clinical research requires analyzing and optimizing the performance of corporate decision makers and study planners versus timelines. The adaptive principle of improving processes based on performance measures should apply to planning and high-level decision making as well as activities between site selection and database lock.

Regulatory Discussions

Regulatory discussions for adaptive programs generally require greater foresight and more precise planning. Exploration of "what-if" scenarios can clarify understanding in regulatory discussions as it does in planning. Since adaptive programs often include quick progression through studies and phases, planners must present regulators with a plan that addresses numerous contingencies and seek a thorough review that accounts for these contingencies. This approach can reduce the likelihood of having to halt development later to address regulatory issues. Use of planning tools such as simulation in advance of regulatory meetings can make discussions more focused and productive.

Regulatory groups will also have to evolve as they recognize the compelling advantages of adaptive methods. The current model of dealing sequentially with each component of a program will have to change to one of specifying acceptable limits at each step and then allowing progression on a "file and go" basis. As with clinical research itself, the relationship between sponsors and regulators must take a more continuous form.

Contingency Planning

Thoughtful what-if discussions have always made valuable contributions to program and study planning. These discussions range from brainstorming to delineating contingencies formally. Discussions usually consider contingencies within a single study. Brainstorming will continue to make important contributions to program planning. However, increased complexity requires that systematic analysis take the leading role. Systematic analysis entails an all-out effort to identify the most likely and significant operational problems in each aspect of the study, from startup through database lock. For maximum benefit, planners should perform this analysis twice: once before writing the plan and a second time afterward. After selection of trial managers, they should provide a third analysis of likely operational problems and roadblocks. If an outside party such as a CRO performs the third operational what-if analysis, the outside perspective will likely increase the number of operational issues anticipated.

Contingency planning also plays a vital role in ongoing management during the trial. Such planning during the trial should make maximum use of the most current data on the state of all significant components of trial operations. This is the best way to identify potential problems and find appropriate solutions. Contingency planning is incomplete without an action plan for responding to each problem that can jeopardize a program's ability to meet timelines or budgetary limitations. Thus, planning should always address contingencies for major operational activities such as enrollment.

The goal of such planning is to arm study managers with a framework that allows them to act quickly in a structured manner rather than counting on the ability to improvise as necessary. While essential, improvisation increases the likelihood of mistakes. The map of contingencies should be as thorough as means and time permit. However, study managers should also recognize that the map is inherently dynamic. At the beginning of the study, an identified set of contingencies should represent something more substantial than an educated guess about which scenarios are most likely and which responses most appropriate. During the study or program, the weight of probability may shift from one scenario to another. It may be necessary to add contingencies that planners overlooked. The spirit of contingency analysis is Bayesian and adaptive: when new information appears, managers must update plans and priorities appropriately.

Planning Tools and Techniques

There may be a temptation to recoil in horror at the sheer complexity that the vast new assortment of possibilities presents—to see so many possibilities as a recipe for chaos. However, powerful planning tools allow more structured thinking about the range of possibilities, defining the most promising and problematic scenarios and recognizing the key decision points. Planning in this manner makes the most of the rich selection of possibilities. This kind of planning may not see the optimal development pathway from the outset, but it defines the way to recognize and pursue the optimal pathway at every point along the way.

Since each clinical program presents a unique set of challenges and the adaptive approach considers addressing these challenges on a wide range of contingencies, there can be no single set of instructions for planning an adaptive study. However, there are tools to simplify considering the range of possibilities and the implications of each. This section introduces two planning tools, decision trees and simulation. Examples show how planning can address design adaptations in early trials that emphasize learning, in later trials that seek to confirm what has already been learned, and in seamless combined-phase trials.

Decision Trees

A decision tree visually shows decisions and their consequences, including outcomes and costs. This tool has the advantage of forcing an explicit, comprehensive exploration of possible outcomes.

Deciding on Sample-Size Reestimation

A decision tree can help in deciding whether to use an adaptive technique. Figure 7-1 shows a decision tree that considers whether a $5 million confirmatory study should use SSRE. This analysis assumes that treating every subject costs about the same. There are three possible outcomes to the study: the magnitude of effect (δ) for the drug being tested is equal to, greater than, or less than the estimate used for determining the initial sample size. For simplicity, this model assumes equal probabilities of a magnitude of effect that is higher than estimated and a magnitude that is lower than estimated. Assuming a 25% probability of a higher magnitude and a 25% probability of a lower magnitude, there is a 50% probability (1–[0.25+0.25]=0.50) that the original estimate will prove correct. We further assume any difference found, whether higher or lower, will differ by 20% from the planning estimate. As a rule of thumb, conventional confirmatory studies build in a 20% enrollment margin for safety. If the results show the observed δ matches or exceeds the planning estimate, the 20% buffer wastes 20% of costs, or $1 million.

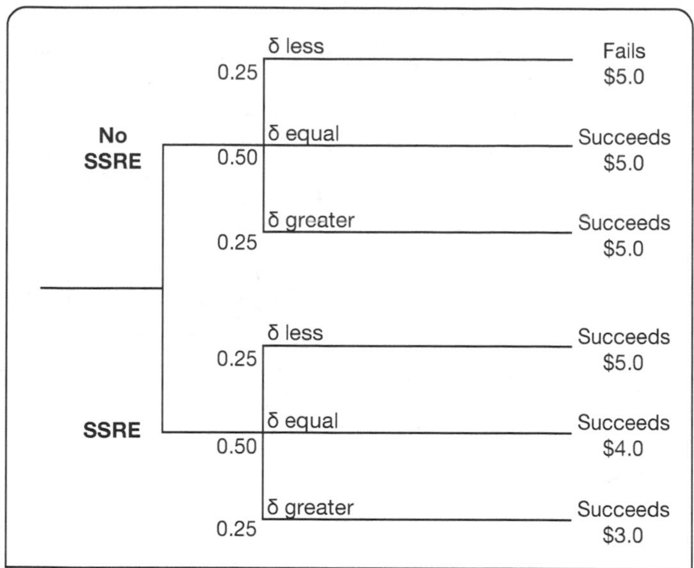

Figure 7-1. Decision tree for evaluating whether to use SSRE in an adaptive study. Possible study outcomes and their respective costs are at far right. Not using SSRE results in uniform cost. However, the topmost arm shows the study failing because of insufficient statistical power.

Without SSRE (no SSRE), the study will cost \$5 million regardless of the observed value of δ. However, in the topmost possibility—an observed δ 20% smaller than estimated—the study will lack the statistical power required to demonstrate a treatment difference. The study will fail and the entire \$5 million investment will go to waste.

The lower half of this tree shows the cost under the same scenarios but with the use of SSRE. If the δ is 20% less than the estimate, the study would reestimate sample size upward, increasing costs to \$5 million but ensuring necessary statistical power. If the δ equals the estimate, SSRE would reduce the sample size by eliminating almost the entire 20% buffer, resulting in a cost of approximately \$4 million. In the most favorable scenario, if the observed δ is 20% greater than the planning estimate, the study would reestimate sample size downward, reducing costs to \$3 million. Thus, as compared to not doing SSRE, the additional cost would be, respectively for the three scenarios, the same (\$5 million), \$1 million less (eliminating the buffer), or \$2 million less (reducing sample size).

Summing the probability-weighted cost of a range of differences between observed and planned effect size shows the penalty for not performing SSRE. Calculating these costs requires multiplying each of the outcomes in the no-SSRE portion by the additional cost as compared to SSRE. For the example discussed above of a 25% probability of higher or lower treatment effect and 50% of its being equal, the probability-weighted total is the sum of each possible outcome, [0.25 × −$5 million]+[0.5 × −$1 million]+[0.25 × −$2 million]= −$2 million. Note that the $5 million loss is due to the failure of the study. The latter two costs represent the additional expense incurred over the SSRE option for addressing different treatment effects. Varying the magnitude of difference between the estimated value of δ used in planning and what is encountered during the study shows the cost of not doing SSRE. The simple conclusion is that the further off planners are from what is actually encountered, the more money is wasted (Figure 7-2). Even when they are found to be spot on in their planning estimates, $1 million is wasted because of the uncertainty inherent in planning estimates and the need to overbuild the study in recognizing that limitation.

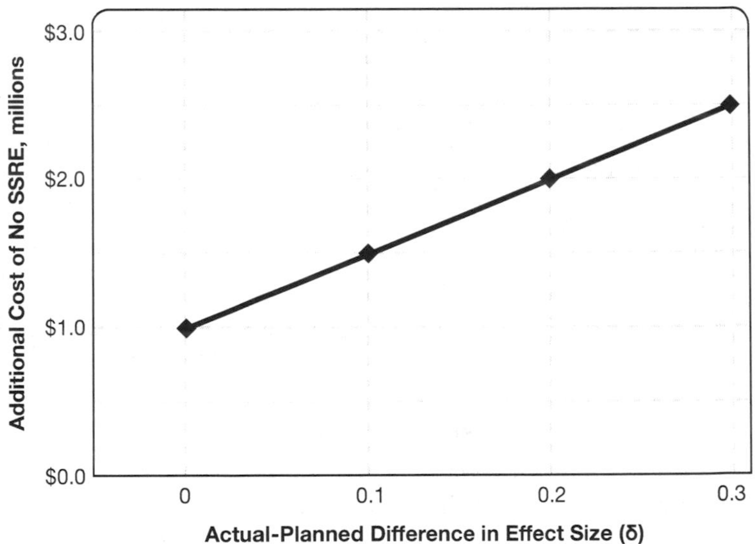

Figure 7-2. The additional cost of not using SSRE, as compared to using SSRE, under scenarios showing effect size differs from the planning estimate.

Decision trees provide insight for planners by allowing them to represent possibilities as nodes in a chart and assign probabilities to each node. Because decision trees use simple probabilities rather than distributions at each branch point, the associated analysis lacks the sophistication of modeling and simulation. However, decision trees clarify relationships among study elements and provide an intuitive sense of how different developments would affect a study.

Specifying and walking through such detailed scenarios force planners to consider how a chain of events might affect important aspects of a study. If the study increased sample size, would the planned number of sites be adequate to recruit the required numbers and types of patients? If the focus of the study narrowed to a responsive subpopulation, would the same type and number of sites be able to recruit enough patients belonging to the subpopulation of interest? A decision tree simplifies estimating the probabilities of each path forward and analyzing the consequences. Modeling tools can help planners explore the importance and likelihood of each possibility. As the study generates data and the status of different aspects of operations becomes clear, updating the probabilities in the decision tree can increase understanding of downstream effects.

Simulation

The FDA has called attention to simulation in the portion of its critical path initiative focused on model-based drug development and in the Agency's draft guidance on end of phase IIa meetings. This draft guidance recommends that sponsors submit simulations in advance to assist the Agency in analyzing next steps.[1] The scope of model-based drug development is sweeping, unifying the dose-response model from discovery to postmarket development. Model-based drug development includes[2]:

- drug and disease modeling;
- exposure-response modeling;
- pharmacometrics.

The availability of a unifying dose-response model encompassing everything from discovery to postmarket development can greatly aid planners of any clinical development program.

However, this section focuses on simulating the practical steps involved in conducting clinical studies. The purpose of such simulations is to explore the effects of different patient response outcomes on the course of the clinical studies and the program as a whole. These simulations focus on the implications of different possible outcomes for the decisions that planners must make in designing studies and the decisions that managers must make in conducting studies efficiently.

Simulation denotes repeated random sampling of a chain of events, with a specified distribution for each event. Simulation is particularly useful for identifying the probabilities of end results and quantifying the influence of each contributing event. Simulations provide more sophisticated analysis than decision trees by using distributions rather than single values for probabilities at each branch point. The power of distributions is to allow attaching a degree of uncertainty to each branch. The use of distributions allows a more nuanced exploration of the possibilities. Simulations often use Gaussian distributions. However, a simulation can use any distribution susceptible to mathematical description, including nonparametric, bimodal, or others.

Uncertainties in Clinical Research

Clinical research has no shortage of uncertainties. Outcomes of clinical trials represent the sum of many component events with varying degrees of uncertainty. Uncertainties exist even at the level of individual patients and doses. Response to repeated outcome measures may vary in the same subject. The precise dose of drugs administered may vary with manufacturing practices and the effectiveness of quality control. Uncertainties also prevail for study populations. For example, rates of patient loss due to dropouts and lost follow-up and rates of actual compliance with regimen vary for different populations and therapeutic areas. Informal assessment of the effects of such an abundance of variations is all but impossible. Simulation makes it practical to quantify the likelihood of different events, outcomes, and downstream effects.

Simulation starts by specifying a model, or mathematical representation of how factors interact, and specifying a distribution for each factor. Simulation is thus a tool for identifying factors in a process, representing interactions among these factors, and exploring the effects of a range of possible inputs on a given outcome. Modern computers can explore the effect of ranges of plausible values for many factors on outcomes tirelessly, thoroughly, and consistently. A modest desktop or laptop computer can run a simulation thousands or even millions of times, often in minutes.

Understanding gleaned from simulations can sometimes identify flawed strategies and opportunities for cost savings that experienced researchers overlook. Humans must still design simulations, supply the input, and judge the results. However, the output of simulations provides valuable input for study planners. A summary of simulation results quantifies the most likely outcomes and the relative importance of each element contributing to the study.

Suitable Areas for Simulation

Simulations have many applications in clinical research. For example, simulations can aid in determining sample size despite uncertainty about contributing factors such as patient dropout rates. Simulations are particularly useful in early clinical development when knowledge of a new drug is limited. For example, simulations can help project drug requirements when there is little basis for forecasting which dosing arms are likely to generate favorable outcomes and continue and which are likely to terminate early.

Indeed, regulators have encouraged the use of simulation as a means of better predicting performance and reducing the high rate of failures in early development. Robert O'Neill, Director of Biostatistics at the FDA's Center for Drug Evaluation and Research, observes:

> *A tool that has been available to statisticians for many years and which is included in some modern software is clinical trial modeling and simulation. Use of such tools in conjunction with data bases or data sets that contain information on disease endpoints, disease progression, patient variability and risk factor or biomarkers should allow for more thorough planning of clinical trials in advance of actually conducting the trials. These tools can be valuable to challenge and explore deviations from the assumptions made for a planned clinical trial, or perhaps for several trials that will be conducted as part of a development program, and these tools can explore before the trial begins the variety of scenarios that may be possible during the actual conduct of the trial. Such modeling and simulations as a tool for better design and interpretation of clinical trials can be considered a modern version of protocol planning that involves much more from statisticians than sample size calculations and other conventional study planning inputs.*[3]

Simulation Tools

A growing range of simulation software is available, including programs available for download without charge. Table 7-1 identifies a sampling of commercial and noncommercial products for simulation as well as related programs for planning and conducting studies given numerous uncertainties.

Table 7-1. Selected Simulation Tools and Related Software

Company/ Institution	Software	Notable Functions	Comments
Cytel	East5, EastAdapt, EastXact	Design of group-sequential, adaptive and fixed-sample-size trials; EastAdapt allows midcourse adjustments for primary and nuisance parameters.	Adaptive module supports three design methods.

Table 7-1. Selected Simulation Tools and Related Software

Company/ Institution	Software	Notable Functions	Comments
Cytel	DoseSim	Response-adaptive randomization, dose selection for phase III	Frequentist and Bayesian approaches; can be integrated with Tourtellotte's supply-chain simulator
Tessella/Berry	Adaptive Trials Simulator	Dose finding and dose selection; predicts outcomes from early responses, allows choice of doses based on estimates of dose response and probability of each dose meeting desired criteria	Bayesian
Tessella	SFT (Supply Forecasting Tool)	Supply forecasting to handle varying allocation based on adaptive dose finding and randomization	Mixture of frequentist and Bayesian techniques
Tourtellotte	TCVisualize	Simulates supply chain	Available integrated with Cytel's DoseSim
CTriSoft	ExpDesign Studio	Supports sequential, multistage, adaptive designs. Adaptive functions include SSRE, adaptive randomization, Bayesian CRM dose finding, adaptive trial simulator	Produces SAS simulation code; bundled with book
ClinBay	Decimaker	Designs and simulates adaptive trials. Bayesian dose response, dose selection, and decision analysis, adaptive randomization	Generates scripts for R statistical environment and OpenBUGs (Bayesian Inference Using Gibbs Sampling)
ADDPLAN GmbH	ADDPLAN 4 (Adaptive Designs—Plans and Analyses)	Design, simulation, and analysis of group sequential studies, including SSRE. Now includes Bayesian elements.	Available by subscription

Table 7-1. Selected Simulation Tools and Related Software

Company/ Institution	Software	Notable Functions	Comments
University of Reading Medical and Pharmaceutical Research Unit	PEST 4 (Planning and Evaluation of Sequential Trials)	Planning and evaluation of sequential trials. Early stopping for presence or absence of treatment difference.	Reads SAS data sets. Available by subscription.
SAS Institute	SAS	The Interactive Matrix Language module provides functions for performing group-sequential tests.	
MD Anderson Biostatistics & Applied Mathematics	ARAND	Adaptive randomization. Outcomes based, up to 10 arms.	Download requires registration.
MD Anderson Biostatistics & Applied Mathematics	Predictive Probability	Bayesian predictive probability analysis	Download requires registration.
Johns Hopkins Oncology Biostatistics	CRM	Dose-finding with CRM method. Bayesian dose-finding based on treatment response.	Downloadable
Johns Hopkins Oncology Biostatistics	Optimal	For simulating optimal two-stage designs. Sample-size reestimation. Allows early termination.	Downloadable
R Project	R Language and Environment	Includes functions for performing group-sequential tests	Downloadable
Christopher Jennison	FORTRAN software for group sequential tests	Includes a variety of programs and routines, including spending function	Downloadable. Supplements book.
Charlie Casper, Oscar A. Perez.	Idbounds.	Performs computation for group-sequential trials including bounds using the Lan-DeMets alpha-spending function approach	Downloadable

Note: Also see "Sources of Simulation Software" at the end of this chapter.

Simulation Step by Step

Simulation involves:

- specifying a model that defines relationships between variables, including chance nodes;
- defining a distribution of plausible values for each chance node;
- running the simulation by sampling each of the variables according to a distribution of values;
- when possible, adjusting the model and distributions to focus on inputs of particular interest.

The simulation program randomly samples each node according to the specified distribution, moves to the next node, and so forth. The result is a set of probabilities for each node and a sum for each "trial." Usually, simulations run until decreases in marginal changes indicate a result with stable final numbers and distributions. Achieving this stability often requires running a simulation hundreds or thousands of times.

The benefit of simulation over the static approach of decision modeling is the ability to run thousands of iterations to generate a distribution of the likelihood of a given outcome. Sensitivity testing, or changing the values of specific variables while holding others constant, provides insight into the degree to which each variable influences the outcome. Example 7-1 shows the use of an open-source trial-simulation tool to aid in determining a study's sample size. This tool can account for uncertainty about effect size, differential dropout, and compliance rates involving unequal allocation ratios in a study involving three subpopulations with different risks.

In a clinical setting, simulations frequently model pharmacokinetics and pharmacodynamics. Increasingly, clinical trials use simulation tools to address predictable issues such as variation between sites and subjects, within-subject variation (especially on complex studies that involve subjective outcomes such as pain and cognition), and magnitude of difference between comparator and drug under development. Simulation can help explore many other factors, such as eliminating or adding subpopulations, ensuring adequate drug and logistics supplies for adaptive trials, analyzing the use of biomarkers, and even implications of the study for portfolio management. Figure 7-3 shows a screen for providing input to a simulation that determines sample size. Figures 7-4 to 7-6 show simulation outputs in three different visual representations.

Example 7-1. Simulation tool for study planning

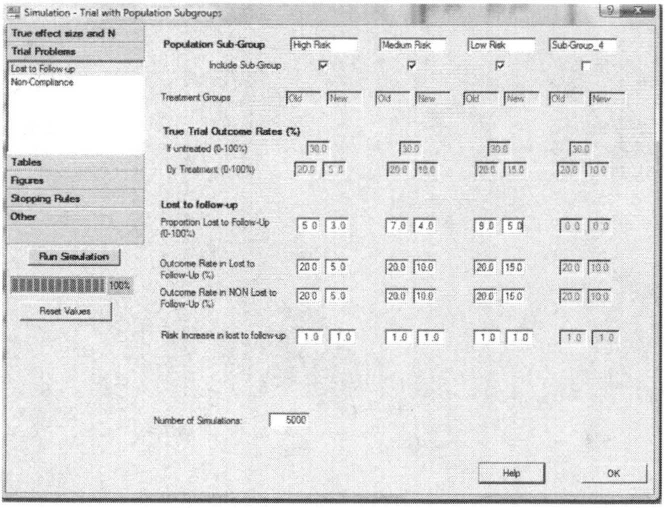

Figure 7-3. Basic sample-size determination on a study involving three subpopulations, including differential rates of loss to follow up in each risk group. Separate screens allow consideration of differential compliance rates in each group.

Screenshots of Clinical Trial Simulator, developed by Eduardo Bergel, David Sacket, and Luz Gibbons on behalf of the PRACTIHC initiative (Pragmatic Randomised Controlled Trials in Health Care) (http://www.practihc.org/).

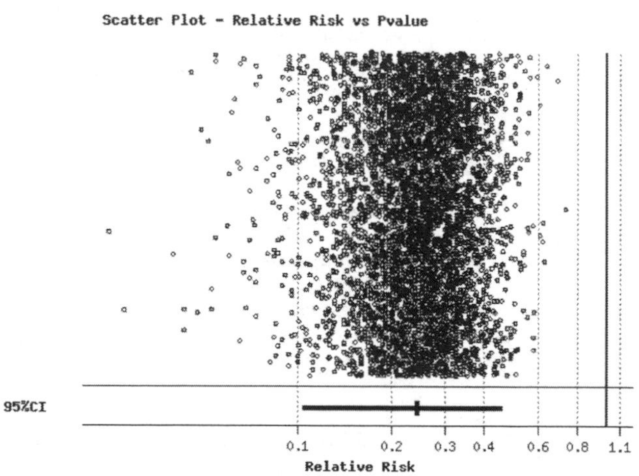

Figure 7-4. Plot of individual outcomes for each of 5,000 simulations. The bottom of the figure shows relative risk and 95% confidence intervals.

Screenshots of Clinical Trial Simulator, developed by Eduardo Bergel, David Sacket, and Luz Gibbons on behalf of the PRACTIHC initiative (Pragmatic Randomised Controlled Trials in Health Care) (http://www.practihc.org/).

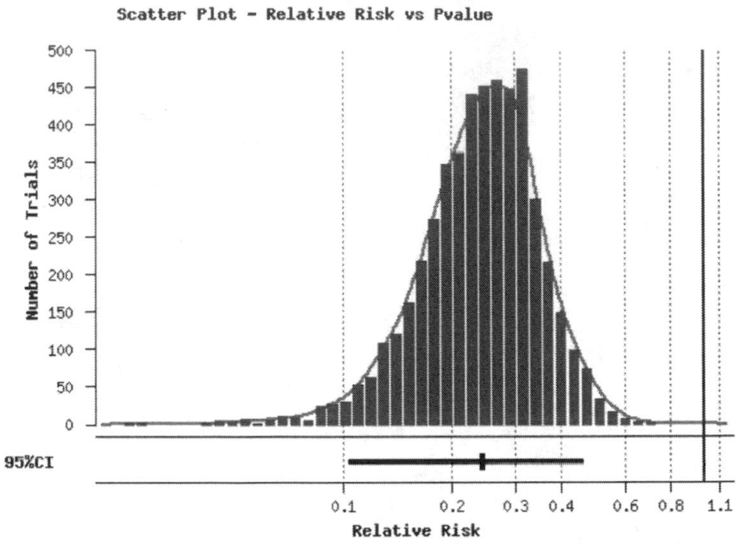

Figure 7-5. Output of simulations in a familiar histogram format.

Screenshots of Clinical Trial Simulator, developed by Eduardo Bergel, David Sacket and Luz Gibbons on behalf of the PRACTIHC initiative (Pragmatic Randomised Controlled Trials in Health Care) (http://www.practihc.org/).

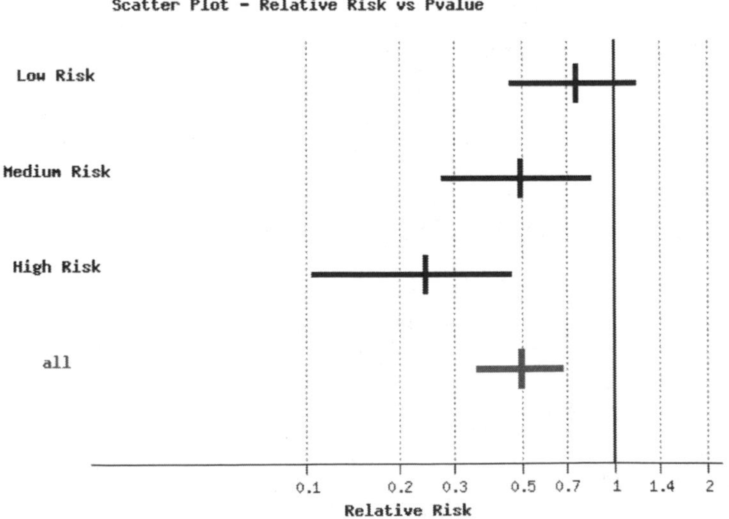

Figure 7-6. Simulation results showing risk and confidence intervals for each subgroup as well as the entire study.

The Limitations of Simulation

If simulation provides value by exploring a range of uncertainties to determine most likely scenarios, the accuracy of the estimates used in a simulation limits that value. The output rests on the relevance and accuracy of input source data, the definition of the model, the selection of key characteristics and behaviors, and inevitable simplifying approximations and assumptions. It is important to remember such limitations when using any software that requests a series of inputs and produces an output without adequately explaining how the transformation takes place.

Example 7-2: Sample-size determination for confirmatory study

Pregnancy was the primary outcome in a noninferiority study of a new type of vaginal contraceptive. Planning sample size required estimates of both rate and timing of pregnancy as well as the patient dropout rate before completion of the two-year observation period. Current regulations require 2,000 woman-months of observation. The question is how many women the study must enroll to meet this requirement.

A simulation considered a range of values that investigators considered plausible. The simulation focused on pregnancy and dropout rates, the two most important parameters affecting months of observation. For these events, the simulation considered both the frequency and the timing. The bimodal distribution of dropouts from contraceptive studies added complexity. The simulation had to account for the pattern of a high dropout rate after study startup, a drop-off, and a second but lower peak.

A series of simulations explored the effects of increasing enrollment in increments of 50, starting at 300, and varying pregnancy rates from 7 to 13 per woman-year explored (Figure 7-4). Researchers started by simulating the results of 5,000 studies, each with a sample size of 300. The simulation calculated total months of exposure for each woman in a single study by sampling predefined distributions for the duration of observation, based on rates of pregnancy, dropout, and loss to follow-up. Then the simulation summed the periods of observation for each woman over 5,000 runs, defining a likely distribution of months of exposure. The simulation repeated the process for larger sample sizes. Investigators used the results to set sample size at 450 women, with an estimated 2.5% probability of 1,986 woman-months, 5% probability of 2,001 woman-months, and 50% probability of 2,079 woman-months. The completed study closely tracked the simulation's projections with 2,100 woman-months of observation and an observed pregnancy rate of 5.1 per 100 woman-months.

300	7	10	11	17	24	25	185	188	215	217	1357	1370	1430	1488	1498	4.0	4.4	7.0	9.8	10.4	7.0	6.4
300	8	12	13	20	27	28	183	185	213	215	1349	1360	1422	1479	1490	4.8	5.3	8.0	10.9	11.6	8.0	6.8
350	7	12	13	20	28	29	217	220	249	252	1592	1603	1668	1729	1743	4.2	4.6	6.9	9.6	10.1	7.0	5.9
350	8	14	16	23	31	33	215	218	247	250	1585	1595	1658	1721	1734	5.0	5.4	8.0	10.8	11.4	8.0	6.4
400	7	15	16	23	31	33	250	253	284	287	1822	1835	1905	1973	1983	4.4	4.8	7.0	9.4	10.0	7.0	5.6
400	8	17	18	26	35	36	247	250	281	284	1817	1829	1896	1962	1976	5.1	5.6	8.0	10.5	11.1	8.0	6.0
450	5	11	12	18	26	27	289	292	324	328	2079	2092	2164	2236	2249	2.9	3.2	5.0	7.0	7.4	5.0	
450	6	14	15	22	30	32	285	289	321	324	2067	2079	2154	2225	2236	3.7	4.0	6.0	8.2	8.6	6.0	
450	7	17	18	26	34	36	282	285	318	322	2057	2072	2145	2216	2228	4.5	4.9	6.9	9.2	9.7	7.0	5.2
450	8	20	21	29	39	40	279	283	316	319	2045	2060	2134	2207	2219	5.3	5.7	7.9	10.4	10.9	8.0	5.6
450	9	23	25	33	43	45	275	279	312	315	2033	2047	2123	2192	2206	6.3	6.6	9.0	11.6	12.1	9.0	5.8
450	10	26	28	37	47	48	272	275	309	312	2021	2036	2111	2181	2194	7.1	7.5	10.0	12.6	13.1	10.0	6.0
450	11	29	31	41	51	53	269	272	306	309	2013	2028	2101	2172	2186	7.8	8.4	10.9	13.8	14.3	11.0	6.5
450	12	33	35	44	55	57	266	269	302	305	1999	2012	2088	2159	2169	8.9	9.4	12.0	14.8	15.4	12.0	6.5
450	13	36	38	48	60	62	262	265	299	303	1986	2001	2079	2151	2165	9.7	10.1	13.0	16.0	16.7	13.0	7.0

Figure 7-7. Simulation for determining sample size (portions). The simulation resulted in setting sample size at 450 women to meet the goal of 2,000 woman-months of observation. The simulation indicated that this sample would allow meeting the goal given nearly all the pregnancy rates in the range explored. Interestingly, total duration of observation showed little sensitivity to pregnancy rate.

Example 7-3: Forecasting drug-supply requirements

Simulations can improve forecasts of the need for drug supplies. In weeks, an adaptive study might move from dose-escalating safety studies to much larger proof-of-concept studies. Inability to package and label the right formulation of the test drug in the right quantities of the right doses and deliver it to the right sites at the right time could cause delays that wipe out potential gains against timelines.

At the outset of an adaptive study, no one knows the quantities and doses that the study will ultimately need. The most cautious approach is to plan supplies of each dosing level for all subjects in each cohort. To improve on such a wasteful approach, studies can use simulations to identify the most likely scenarios. For example, suppose a dose-finding study starts with once-daily doses of 10, 30, 50, 100, and 200 mg. The study's goal is to reduce the number of arms to no more than two after two months of observation and to a single dose suitable for confirmatory studies within four months. However, manufacturing the drug takes three weeks. Quality testing, packaging, and distribution to sites take one week each. Thus, lead time for drug supplies is seven weeks. A conventional approach would package doses of 10 and 50 mg and meet dosing needs with multiple-pill combinations, as well as arranging two matching placebos to prevent patients from knowing which dose they are receiving.

To determine the most likely scenario, simulations can use estimates of the likely outcomes weighted according to previous knowledge. The simulation can then update these estimates based on data collected as the study proceeds. Such a simulation might include: (1) the probability of safety issues based on limited human data or extrapolation from animal data; (2) varied results for efficacy, also based on prior human or animal results; (3) estimated drug manufacturing lead times that include quality control; and (4) estimated lead times for different forms of packaging.

A decision tree provides a useful starting point for creating a simulation. The decision tree specifies each possible outcome and points along the way, both chance events and decisions. Adaptive methods allow continually updating the probability of chance events with new information. Decision events represent choices such as whether to maintain, increase, or decrease the number of patients in each arm and whether to continue or end each dosing arm. Adaptive studies, especially for dose finding, may allow ending nonperforming arms when data suggests futility. However, drug availability limits possible decisions. Ordering full supplies for each arm can be both wasteful and expensive. Researchers must try to ensure manufacturing and packaging of enough study supplies while minimizing waste. The option to expand or reduce the number of patients in each dosing arm thus requires considering the speed and reliability of decision making about dosing arms and the supplier's ability to meet changing needs. In a further complication, studies can sometimes repackage existing supplies.

Study planners need to weigh the benefit of reducing lead time for ordering supplies against the likely higher cost of obtaining different quantities on short notice. If costs are high, the wise course might be suspending enrollment to await production of additional supplies. If costs are low, it makes more sense to invest in manufacturing 10- and 50-mg doses before the study begins, thus reducing lead times.

A conventional approach to providing supplies for a 60-day dosing study that included arms taking 10-, 30-, 50-, 100-, and 200-mg doses, with each subject taking four tablets per day, would require 240 10-mg tablets and 240 dummy tablets to provide doses of 10 and 30 mg. Similarly, doses of 50, 100, and 200 mg would require active 50-mg tablets and dummy tablets in quantities of 60 and 180, 120 and 120, and 240 and 0, respectively. A study with 50 subjects per arm would require 12,000 10-mg tablets, 21,000 50-mg tablets, and 27,000 dummy tablets.

Simulation could provide estimates of the number of pills of each dose based on the likelihood and distribution of the probability of each arm. For example, a probability of the 10-mg arm might be felt unlikely and assigned a probability of 0.3, with a normal distribution and standard deviation of 0.1. Probabilities and distributions could similarly be assigned each dose, to produce a distribution of estimates of the likelihood of the number of each tablet dose level. An adaptive approach updates probabilities as data accumulates during the study, with decision cutoffs based on lead times for the manufacture and packaging of supplies either for the same or for a subsequent study. For example, a six-month drug lead time as the critical path to the next study means that probabilities of different dosing arms being continued could be updated six months before the planned initiation of the next study. Depending on the nature of the information available at that time, the decision might be to go ahead with the production of certain doses. Alternatively, the decision might be to postpone the following study while awaiting even better estimates.

As the study progresses, the likelihood that each dosing arm will continue changes based on efficacy and safety data. For example, the study might use a simulation to examine different distributions of probabilities for success of dosing arms of 10, 30, 50, 100, and 200 mg. The study would use the output of the simulation, with updates based on study data, to adjust supply orders to meet the needs of the arms most likely to continue.

Conclusions

Adaptive programs require greater planning because of their long-term perspective and the close interplay between operational and strategic elements. Careful planning is essential if adaptive research is to provide greater control of studies and programs, dynamically allocate resources to activities that produce the greatest return, and minimize or eliminate dead time. Modeling and simulation are important tools that help assess the uncertainty inherent in clinical development. These tools can provide illuminating input for decision making.

Such a comprehensive and painstaking approach to planning reduces the likelihood of major surprises. Managers can sleep better knowing that they are less likely to encounter a completely unforeseen situation in midstudy. Managing studies in accordance with such carefully thought-out plans is superior to the less reflective conventional approach that requires dealing with issues as they arise based on whatever information happens to be available. The greatest benefit of the detailed planning process for adaptive studies and programs is giving managers the ability to understand how a study is progressing, select appropriate responses based on previously defined plans, and optimize the course of development in response to the realities encountered. The more rigorous approach to planning gives managers greater control over the fate of development programs.

Superior planning cannot transform an ineffective drug into a marketable treatment. However, better planning can reduce timelines and costs, weed out poor candidates earlier, allow a deeper understanding of drugs under test, and allow faster exploitation of successes. Study and program managers will understand that such benefits far outweigh the effort required for more detailed and precise planning.

References

1 U.S. Department of Health and Human Services, Food and Drug Administration, Center for Drug Evaluation and Research (CDER). Washington. Guidance for industry end-of-phase 2A meetings. Sept 2008. Available from: http://www.fda.gov/cder/Guidance/8297dft.htm.

2 Stanksi DR. Model-based drug development: a Critical Path opportunity. Feb 25, 2004. Available from: http://www.fda.gov/oc/initiatives/criticalpath/stanski/stanski.html.

3 O'Neill RT. FDA's Critical Path Initiative: a perspective on contributions of biostatistics. Biom J. 2006;48(4):559–64.

Sources of Simulation Software

Chang M. Classical and adaptive clinical trial designs using ExpDesign Studio. New York: Wiley Interscience; 2008.

http://biostatistics.mdanderson.org/SoftwareDownload/SingleSoftware.aspx?Software_Id=62.

http://biostatistics.mdanderson.org/SoftwareDownload/SingleSoftware.aspx?Software_Id=10.

http://www.cancerbiostats.onc.jhmi.edu/software.cfm.

http://randomization.org/downloads.htm.

http://people.bath.ac.uk/mascj/book/programs/general.

Jennison C, Turnbull B. Group sequential methods with application to clinical trials. Boca Raton, FL: Chapman & Hall/CRC; 1999.

http://cran.r-project.org/web/packages/ldbounds/.

Comprehensive R Archive Network sites listed at: http://www.r-project.org.

— Chapter 8 —

Statistics and Decision Making in Adaptive Research

The *frequentist* approach to statistics has long dominated clinical research. Trial design, data analysis, managerial decision making, and regulatory review all rely largely on frequentist methods. However, interest in the *Bayesian* approach to statistics is growing, especially in adaptive studies. Differences between frequentist and Bayesian statistics have important implications for the design and evaluation of adaptive studies and programs.

The Frequentist Approach

The frequentist approach to statistics provides valuable structure for designing experiments and analyzing results. The frequentist approach starts by postulating a *null hypothesis* of no difference between treatments or interventions. The familiar *p*-value measures the probability that, if the hypothesis were true, the results of many repetitions of the same experiment would be as extreme or more extreme than those observed in a given study. The name *frequentist* comes from assessing the frequency of getting a result as or more extreme than the results observed.

In practice, the frequentist approach to study design and interpretation is straightforward. Planners define the null hypothesis and specify the desired level of significance (traditionally $p<0.05$) and statistical power, or ability to detect a difference. After the study is complete, biostatisticians calculate the *p*-value. If $p<0.05$, the results are termed statistically significant. Researchers reject the null hypothesis and treat the results as though the evidence collected in the trial shows that the drug works. However, this inference about the meaning of the *p*-value is wrong. The drug may work, but the frequentist statistical methods do not directly address the question of whether the evidence collected in the study shows that the null hypothesis is false and the alternative hypothesis is true.

Many drug researchers misunderstand the meaning of frequentist significance tests. Many who do understand the meaning of frequentist significance tests nevertheless draw stronger conclusions than the strict interpretation of such tests justifies. In both cases, the main reason is the lack of an alternative approach to statistics. Although frequentist statistics have dominated for decades, widespread confusion exists about the underlying principles and the meaning of frequentist parameters cited for the results of specific clinical trials. Addressing this confusion starts by distinguishing between what frequentist methods actually tell us about the results of a specific clinical trial and how, in practice, we use frequentist methods to review trial data and make decisions about whether new drugs work.

What Frequentist Results Say about the Results of a Clinical Study

There is little wonder that people misinterpret *p*-values. The definition itself seems anything but straightforward: the probability of observing in many repetitions of the same trial a result as or more extreme than that observed, assuming that there is no difference between the two treatments. If you have to reread this sentence, and especially if it remains unclear after a second reading, take a number. The indirect nature of *p*-values makes them less than intuitive. The *p*-values are not derived from data collected during a study. They are a very indirect way of providing a basis for assessing not the truth of a hypothesis but the plausibility of the results of a study. Even researchers who routinely rely on *p*-values often misunderstand their meaning. David Salsburg, former head of statistics for Pfizer, addresses the confusion about *p*-values as follows:

> [A *p*-value] is a theoretical probability associated with the observations under conditions that are most likely false. It has nothing to do with reality. It is an indirect measurement of plausibility. It is not the probability that we would be wrong to say the drug works. It is not the probability of any kind of error. It is not the probability that the patient will do as well on the placebo as on the drug.[1]

Salsburg's phrase *nothing to do with reality* is perhaps not what clinical researchers attempting to demonstrate the effectiveness of a new drug want to hear about *p*-values. Despite common usage, a *p*-value of <0.05 does *not* imply rejection of the null hypothesis of no difference between the test drug and the comparator. Such a *p*-value does not confirm the alternative hypothesis that the new drug works. Although *p*-values quantify probabilities, the probabilities do not apply to the likelihood that a new drug is effective. Thus, a *p*-value of 0.05 does not indicate that study data demonstrates a 5% probability of no difference between test drug and comparator, nor does it imply that the data shows a 95% probability that the test drug is effective. In the frequentist way of thinking, a hypothesis is either true or false. There is either a 100% probability that the hypothesis is true and a 0% probability that the hypothesis is false or the reverse. There is no way to speak about probabilities in between.

Confusion about Statistical Power

Another common source of confusion about frequentist methods is the now standard approach to hypothesis testing descended from the ideas of Fisher, Neyman, and Egon Pearson. This form of hypothesis testing states two hypotheses: the null hypothesis of no treatment effect and an alternative hypothesis that there is a treatment effect. The approach quantifies the risk of a false-positive or false-negative result—concluding that there is no difference between the test drug and the comparator when there is a difference or that there is a difference when there is none. By assuming that a hypothesis is true, this method can calculate rates for both types of error. However, like *p*-values, the rates are those to be expected in many repetitions of the same trial.

Today's standard approach to hypothesis testing includes the concept of statistical *power*. The power is the probability of rejecting the null hypothesis for a specific value of an alternative hypothesis. The purpose of this measure is to ensure the ability to detect a difference between the test drug and a comparator if a difference exists. However, this standard approach to hypothesis testing says nothing about the truth of the null hypothesis or the alternative hypothesis based on the data collected in a single trial. The Neyman-Pearson paper introducing the approach suggested that no individual experiment could establish the truth of a hypothesis.[2] Therefore, the approach focuses on limiting the incidence of errors in repetitions of the trial over the long term. Learning the truth of a separate hypothesis in a separate trial is not within the scope of frequentist techniques.

Using Frequentist Results to Make Decisions Based on Individual Trials

Now for the great paradox of frequentist statistics: although frequentist methods say nothing about the truth of a hypothesis in any specific trial, standard practice uses frequentist methods to do exactly that. In the real world, sponsors and regulators must assess whether new drugs work. Sponsors conduct studies for this express purpose. Frequentist statistical methods serve as tools for assessing the truth of the hypotheses in each separate trial. If a trial has adequate statistical power and shows a treatment difference and the results produce a *p*-value of 0.05 or less, sponsors and regulators conclude that the individual trial has demonstrated the effectiveness of the test drug. There is seldom an acknowledgement that the *p*-value of 0.05 indicates only that the data collected in the specific trial is unlikely to be the result of chance. Sponsors and regulators seldom emphasize that the low false-positive and false-negative rates refer not to the current trial but to many putative repetitions of the same trial. In keeping with the goal of the individual trial and the need to make decisions, sponsors and regulators act as though favorable frequentist numbers show that there is very little chance of error in the results of the specific trial. Indeed, they act as though a study with a *p*-value <0.05 shows that the probability that the new drug does not work is less than 5%.

In announcing the approval of a new drug, nobody emphasizes the true long-term reference of the time-honored 95% significance level of the frequentist approach, the *p*-value of 0.05 that has become the Holy Grail of billion-dollar development programs. Certainly, nobody reminds shareholders and physicians that the frequentist methods used do not address the central question about the current trial of the new drug: Does the data collected in the specific trial show a high probability that the drug works? Why, then, do the drug industry and its regulators use frequentist methods to judge whether the results of individual trials demonstrate a high probability that a new drug works? The answer is simple. For decades, frequentist statistics have performed this important function because there has been no alternative.

By now, it should be clear that the confusion about frequentist statistics arises from the incongruence between the questions that frequentist methods actually answer and their routine use to answer questions that are more specific and urgent. This is not to deny the value of frequentist methods or to discount their service to the drug industry. Few would deny that indirect frequentist measures of plausibility have proved a valuable way to use the results of individual studies to judge the effectiveness of new drugs. Nevertheless, the absence of a direct way to measure evidence, or judge truth, in an individual experiment must be seen as an important limitation in a scientific culture that does, in fact, use individual experiments for that purpose.

The frequent misinterpretation of frequentist statistics teaches another important lesson. Over the years, statisticians have tried mightily to counter the misinterpretation of a 95% significance level as the probability that a new drug is effective. However, their meticulous explanations of frequentist methods have proved no match for the tendency to find a predictive probability where there is none. The strength and pervasiveness of this tendency show that many people, including researchers, yearn for a more direct statistical approach—an approach that does use data collected during a study to assess the probability that a new drug works. As statistical methods that satisfy this yearning become more prevalent, statisticians will lead easier lives.

Other Issues with Frequentist Methods

In practice, the frequentist approach to statistics has characteristics that complicate its use in adaptive studies. Perhaps the greatest such limitation concerns support for incremental learning. Frequentist methods are fundamentally retrospective. There is a penalty in error rates for interim looks at data. Although statisticians have developed frequentist techniques to allow for sample-size reestimation based on actual study data, these methods raise issues about preserving alpha—in plain words, ensuring that multiple looks do not lead to erroneous results. With frequentist methods, one or two interim looks may be workable. However, the lack of a convenient, ever-present mechanism for incorporating new information during a study can increase costs and decrease efficiency. Continuous learning and frequentist methods do not make a happy couple.

The frequentist approach at times seems poorly suited to addressing the high level of uncertainty that is inherent in drug development. Study results often reveal that planning estimates of key parameters such as magnitude of treatment effect miss the mark. Statistical methods that simplify correcting such estimates during a study have great appeal. Frequentist methods do not always provide the most convenient mechanisms for handling such surprises.

The frequentist approach also has difficulty adjusting hypotheses. The approach is best suited to testing a single, unchanging hypothesis for the duration of a study and analyzing data at the end. Unstinting focus on a single hypothesis has strong appeal in the final stages of drug development. The goal of late-stage studies is to confirm findings from previous studies, providing a definitive assessment of a test drug's efficacy and safety. Sponsors and regulators need a yes or no answer. The traditional drug development process holds that a study using the frequentist approach either provides statistically significant evidence in favor of a specific hypothesis about the new drug or does not—yes or no. The ability to provide such a definitive answer has helped make the frequentist approach the basis for decision making by regulators and researchers. However, rigid adherence to a single hypothesis throughout a study is less useful in early development when uncertainty about how a new drug or device may affect test subjects is often great. Such a high degree of uncertainty makes it difficult to formulate an appropriate hypothesis to test. Research can become a trial-and-error approach in which each trial is literally a new trial with a new hypothesis. Such a sequence of trials is unlikely to be the most efficient way to acquire information in early development.

Although sometimes a strength, providing a sharp cut-off between yes and no can sometimes be a weakness with frequentist methods as practiced. The precipitous cutoff between significance and nonsignificance, with a *p*-value of 0.05 as the razor's edge, can make a profound difference, like the few shillings in David Copperfield that make the difference between enjoying freedom and going to debtors' prison[3]:

> Annual income twenty pounds, annual expenditure nineteen six, result happiness. Annual income twenty pounds, annual expenditure twenty pound ought and six, result misery.

Pharma companies and their shareholders have lost more than a few shillings because of this sharp differentiation between success and failure. Few experienced researchers have escaped the experience of reaching the end of a frequentist study only to find a near miss on the required statistical significance. Researchers can only ask themselves where they went wrong in planning the study. Although the use of confidence intervals rather than single values of an outcome measure helps to address this issue, the basic structure of the frequentist approach, along with its assessment of significance, remains unchanged.

Another limitation of frequentist methods is that both magnitude of effect and sample size influence *p*-values. A significant *p*-value can result from a large magnitude of effect and a small sample size, but the same *p*-value can result from a small magnitude of effect and a large sample size. Studies with small sample sizes typical of early development have difficulty achieving desired *p*-values unless treatment differences are great. Often the consequence is increasing the size of early studies beyond what alternative methods require for the purposes of early development.

The Bayesian Approach

The Bayesian approach to statistics bases its conclusions on the evidence observed, updating an assessment of the probability that a hypothesis is true with each piece of data. Thomas Bayes, a mathematician and minister, identified the fundamental principle of this approach in a paper published in 1763, two years after his death.[4]

Over the years, but especially in the 20th century, mathematicians and statisticians have expanded and strengthened the mathematical foundations of the approach that Bayes' idea suggested.[5]

The Bayesian method examines the data collected and attempts to determine its import: "Given the data that we have collected, what can we infer?" Starting statistical analysis with the data collected in a study hardly seems a radical idea. However, the analysis proceeds in the opposite direction from frequentist methods. The frequentist approach begins by asking, "Given the hypothesis, how likely is the data we have collected?"

With the Bayesian approach, the greater the amount of confirming evidence collected during a study, the higher the degree of belief in the hypothesis; the greater the amount of evidence collected to the contrary, the higher the degree of disbelief. The Bayesian approach has intuitive appeal because it appears to mimic the thought processes of a rational being in daily life. Rational people base judgments and decisions on a combination of previous experience and new information acquired up to the point of making a judgment or decision. Despite such appealing characteristics, the difficulty of the calculations required to solve many problems using Bayesian methods was until recent decades a severe barrier to widespread acceptance. Access to great computing power at low cost has now swept that barrier aside.

Prior Distributions

Because the Bayesian approach relies on incremental modification of an existing belief, the first step is specifying an initial belief. The initial belief is a probability distribution. The distribution may be uniform or "noninformative," assigning equal probability to every possible answer. However, if strong and highly relevant information exists, the Bayesian approach can take advantage of the information by incorporating it in the prior distribution. The prior distribution could reflect data from similar studies of similar drugs or from a completed study of the same test drug. Once established, the initial distribution changes with each new piece of information. The greater the amount of data collected, the more the collected data overwhelms the initial distribution.

The Bayesian approach deals with the unknown parameter as a random variable. With more data, the distribution reflects a higher probability that the random variable falls within a range. If the probability that the value falls within a certain range increases to 95%, that corresponds to the intuitive sense of 95% confidence that the true value does fall within that range. It is important to be mindful of how greatly this approach to developing confidence in study results differs from the frequentist approach. Because the frequentist approach considers key parameters as unknown constants, the intuitive sense of confidence in the result of a study using frequentist statistics is more elusive. It does not make sense to speak of a distribution of values for a parameter that is a constant. Although the 95% confidence level in frequentist statistics concerns a probability distribution, the distribution reflects not trial data, but results that would be expected if the trial were to be repeated many times. The 95% confidence level of frequentist statistics does not express confidence that the value of a parameter for the test drug falls within a range.

How Bayesian Statistics Works

Bayes' famous equation quantified a rule for updating or revising the strength, or likelihood, of a belief, such as a belief about the truth of a hypothesis, in light of new evidence.

Bayes' theorem has three components:

- a subjective starting point that expresses a "best guess" of the hypothesis being true before collecting any data (*the prior probability*);
- an element through which data speak by comparing the fit against the null and alternate hypotheses (*the Bayes factor*); and
- the updated probability that the null hypothesis is true (*posterior or conditional odds*).

Prior probability X **Bayes factor** = **Posterior conditional odds**

where the Bayes factor is

$$\frac{\textit{Probability of data, given null hypothesis}}{\textit{Probability of data, given alternative hypothesis}}$$

or a comparison of how well the two hypotheses predict the data. Stated slightly differently, Bayes expresses the probability of the hypothesis given the data [$P(\text{hyp} \mid \text{data})$] as the product of the probability of data given the hypothesis [$P(\text{data} \mid \text{hyp})$] and the probability of the hypothesis [$P(\text{hyp})$]. Mathematically, this is expressed as

$$P(A \mid B) = \frac{P(B \mid A)P(A)}{P(B)}$$

where

- $P(A)$ is the *prior probability* (also called *marginal probability*) of A. This does not take into account any information on B;
- $P(A \mid B)$ is the *conditional probability* of A, given B. It is also called the *posterior probability* because it depends upon the value of B;
- $P(B \mid A)$ is the conditional probability of B given A;
- $P(B)$ is the *prior* or *marginal probability* of B and acts as a normalizing constant to keep the probability between 0 and 1.0.

Bayesian Statistics in the Real World

With increasing availability of computing power, researchers have applied Bayesian methods to a wide range of problems. The goal has not always been to use Bayesian methods, nor has the choice of Bayesian methods always been conscious or intentional. To help break the German Enigma codes during World War II, Alan Turing invented a technique to guess the settings of an Enigma machine by statistical examination of the text of the messages containing the settings. The Enigma machine's settings determined how a series of rotors—disks that electrically substituted one character for another—encrypted text before transmission and decrypted text after transmission. The sender and receiver of a message had to use the same rotors in the same sequence with the same settings. Blessed with unique access to computing power in its infancy, the code breakers at Bletchley Park could employ techniques such as the one that Turing developed to determine the Enigma settings that were in use. The technique in this instance used what Turing called a "factor in favor of a hypothesis." This factor was the Bayes factor. However, Turing was unaware of this and had invented the technique independently. Turing was simply trying to solve a pressing problem and developed a method that worked.[6]

The Bayesian approach has helped determine authorship of *The Federalist Papers* by examining use of specific words and phrases,[7] projected election results from partial returns,[8] managed investment portfolios, and optimized search-engine results and spam filters. Bayesian statistics play a growing role in the sciences, including physics, robotics, and environmental analysis. In the health sciences, Bayesian statistics perform medical risk assessments and diagnostics for conditions such as breast cancer. To take one example of how Bayesian methods work in practical applications, spam filters attempt to identify unwanted e-mail based on certain characteristics. At the outset, a spam filter may assume that certain characteristics identify e-mail as spam or may begin with a noninformative prior distribution, regarding all e-mail as equally likely to be spam or not. As user feedback identifies spam over time, the Bayesian filter refines associations of e-mail characteristics with spam and increases accuracy in identifying spam without user intervention.[9]

Bayesian Methods in Clinical Research

Although clinical research was once entirely frequentist, Bayesian statistics is finding favor in a variety of areas, including the well-established continual reassessment method of dose finding. In a pharmaceutical context, we start by hypothesizing that drug B can produce a desired outcome (say, a cure) with a given probability [$P(A)$]. Suppose we launch a study in which we give patients drug B and, after a given time, we observe whether they are cured [$P(B \mid A)$]. If conducted using the typical frequentist approach, the study determines a sample size in advance based on estimates of parameters such as treatment effect and then continues until it has collected all the data required to test the hypothesis. With a limited number of exceptions, there is usually little or no knowledge of accumulating results along the way. A study using Bayesian statistics might, as each patient reaches an endpoint, update the probability of cure $P(B \mid A)$ in patients treated with drug B. A Bayesian study might reach its endpoint when there is sufficient confidence—a high posterior probability—that drug B does or does not work. The endpoint might come when the prior odds, a best assessment or neutral value that has been updated along the way, reaches a prespecified value (normally >0.95) or a predetermined number of subjects has been evaluated without achieving that endpoint. For example, in oncology studies, one endpoint might be survival to a given point, and another might be disease progression. The Bayesian approach thus allows updating a best estimate of efficacy as each new piece of knowledge becomes available (Figure 8-1).

Comparing Bayesian and Frequentist Methods

For clinical trials, Bayesian statistical methods provide important benefits, including:

- more directly addressing the central question of a study;
- producing probability estimates of study results;
- providing predictive probabilities that preview study results and aid midcourse decision making;
- providing a more intuitive basis for decision making;

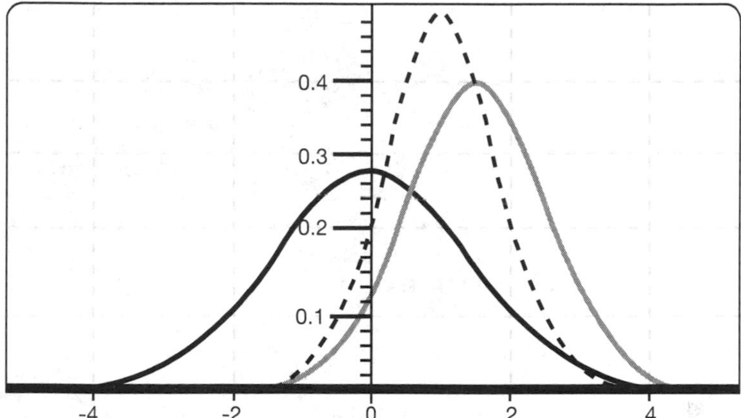

Figure 8-1. Bayesian updating, starting with the prior distribution (black line), updating with new data (gray line), producing an updated estimate or posterior distribution (dashed line). The prior distribution indicates that the value lies between +4 and −4, most likely between +2 and −1, with a best estimate of 0. The new data favors values between 0 and +3. The posterior combines these two sources of data to suggest that the most likely value lies around 1, and values greater than 3 and less than 1 are highly unlikely.

- if desired, incorporating existing knowledge from multiple sources and producing results that take the additional knowledge into account;
- incorporating a distribution (range of values) rather than a single estimate, allowing data input and providing output that is more nuanced and more reflective of the uncertain state of actual knowledge;
- facilitating the use of decision criteria in adaptive trials that include flexible dosing and patient-allocation ratios (for example, response-adaptive randomization);
- relying on a single formula, Bayes' rule, for updating probabilities, with the full range of sample sizes.

Table 8-1 summarizes some key differences between frequentist and Bayesian statistics.

Table 8-1. Contrasting frequentist and Bayesian statistical methods.

	Frequentist	Bayesian
Nature of probability	Probability is a limit of long-run frequency in a large number of repeatable events	Personal degree of belief relevant to any occurrence about which we are uncertain
Nature of parameters	Parameters are unknown fixed values reflecting a population and are estimated through sampling	Parameters are represented by a probability distribution
Prior information	Not utilized, though may be considered in design phase	Explicitly used as a starting point (defining probability distribution)
Interim analyses	Inferences require adjustment to minimize risk of false positive	No adjustment needed
Interim predictions	Conditional power	Predictive probability
Nature of inference	Does not make statements about parameters, although it appears to	Makes direct probability statements about parameters
Interpretation of test results	• Point estimates • *p*-values or confidence intervals	• Parameter distributions are updated after observing data • Credible intervals
Example of interpretation	• "I reject this hypothesis at the 5% level of significance." • In 5% of samples where the hypothesis is true, it will be rejected; says nothing about the current sample	• "The probability that this hypothesis is true is 0.05." • The statement applies on the basis of the observed data

Note: There are exceptions to the generalizations in this table.

Prior Distributions

The ability of the Bayesian approach to incorporate information as a starting point—the prior distribution—strikes some people as an advantage and others as a disadvantage. The prior distribution may summarize knowledge from expert opinion, from posterior probabilities of previous human studies, or even from animal work. Some critics consider the selection of any prior distribution as inherently subjective. On the other hand, the Bayesian school that mandates using the noninformative (uniform) distribution as the prior goes by the name "objective Bayesian analysis."

With a commitment to select prior distributions that are either noninformative or based on the best available hard information, the "subjectivity" of the Bayesian approach bears little resemblance to the ordinary meaning of the term. Whatever the prior, the key question is how much data is required to marginalize its influence. With enough data, the data will converge on the same posterior probability regardless of the prior. With a skeptical prior (one that assumes a drug does not work), it will simply take longer to demonstrate that an effective drug does work. A noninformative prior will get to the same point sooner. A prior that incorporates previous work indicating that the drug is effective will take even less data and reach a conclusion still sooner.

In practice, a Bayesian confirmatory study would begin with a noninformative prior, such as a uniform distribution, where any result has the same likelihood as any other. The purpose of noninformative priors is precisely to minimize the effect of the prior distribution on inferences drawn from the study. Furthermore, because the Bayesian approach makes prior probabilities explicit, researchers can always explore the effect of using different priors to analyze the same data through techniques such as sensitivity testing.

Finally, subjectivity can creep into studies regardless of methodology. Studies using frequentist methods cannot exclude subjectivity from the selection of hypotheses, estimates of parameters, and assumptions about models.

Although regulatory guidance on the selection of prior distributions is limited, the increasing use of Bayesian methods, especially in device trials, reflects acceptance of a range of priors. Current guidance for the device industry states[10]:

> Good prior information is often available for a medical device; for example, from earlier studies on previous generations of the device or from studies overseas. These studies can often be used as prior information because the mechanism of action of medical devices is typically physical, making the effects local and not systemic. Local effects are often predictable from prior information when modifications to a device are minor.
>
> Bayesian methods may be controversial when the prior information is based mainly on personal opinion (often derived by elicitation methods). The methods are often not controversial when the prior information is based on empirical evidence such as prior clinical trials. Since sample sizes are typically small for device trials, good prior information can have greater impact on the analysis of the trial and thus on the FDA decision process.

Regardless of methodology, the important thing in clinical research is to focus, insofar as data allows, on determining the truth about the safety and efficacy of new drugs. The judgment is ultimately medical. Statistical analysis of the data collected informs such a judgment, and standards for the use of statistics set the rules. However, the role of medical expertise does not begin and end at the planning stage. Whether the analysis is Bayesian or frequentist, medical judgment remains the ultimate test.

The Pharma Context

Learning and Confirming

Although both frequentist and Bayesian methods provide powerful tools that are used for systematically assessing the truth of a hypothesis, the difference in approach can have pronounced effects on the perception and use of study results. The supposed Bayesian weakness of assigning a prior distribution affects the perception of results from studies that use Bayesian statistics. For some people, concerns about the indirect basis for frequentist inferences affect the perception of the results of studies that use frequentist methods.

As a practical matter, dependence on stating a prior distribution has limited the use of Bayesian methods to date primarily to the early learning phases of clinical research in which uncertainty is great and the goal is to assess safety or define an optimal dose for confirmatory testing. Bayesian methods address the challenges of early development well by identifying posterior probabilities and credible intervals. The high failure rate of drugs in late-stage studies may indicate that early trials using other methods have sometimes done a poor job of dose selection.

Bayesian statistics and adaptive methods hold the promise of more effective decision making about effective and safe doses and earlier recognition that a drug is ineffective or unsafe. Using Bayesian methods to achieve these goals is far more efficient than reaching the same conclusion after a large, costly, late-stage study. Bayesian statistics and adaptive techniques are already changing research and will continue to do so as experience accumulates and statistical methodology evolves.

Ethical and Operational Issues

Bayesian and frequentist approaches allowing midcourse looks can present different ethical considerations as well as different operational implications for ensuring the exclusion of bias. The range of ethical considerations can change, especially with life-threatening health conditions, because a midcourse look may reveal that one test dose appears to be effective, with markedly fewer deaths among patients allocated to that treatment arm, while an arm that gives patients a comparator experiences a much higher rate of deaths. The obvious ethical consideration concerns continuing to allocate patients to the comparator arm knowing that such an assignment increases the likelihood of death for those patients.

Operational considerations change with the possibility of midcourse corrections. The acquisition of more knowledge earlier in the trial increases the risk of exposing members of the study team to information that could allow the introduction of bias; Chapter 9 discusses this and other considerations in establishing a reliable platform for conducting adaptive trials. The expanded range of ethical and operational considerations presents new challenges but does not change the fundamental goal: to make unbiased assessments of the efficacy of new treatments while doing the utmost to protect test subjects.

Regulatory Considerations

Regulators have been cautiously receptive to Bayesian methods. Together with Johns Hopkins University, the FDA has conducted a workshop, "Can Bayesian Approaches to Studying New Treatments Improve Regulatory Decision-Making?"[11] The FDA has also issued guidance documents on the use of Bayesian statistics in device studies[10]:

> When good prior information on clinical use of a device exists, the Bayesian approach may enable FDA to reach the same decision on a device with a smaller-sized or shorter-duration pivotal trial.
>
> The Bayesian approach may also be useful in the absence of informative prior information. First, the approach can provide flexible methods for handling interim analyses and other modifications to trials in midcourse (e.g., changes to the sample size or changes in the randomization scheme). Second, the Bayesian approach can be useful in complex modeling situations where a frequentist analysis is difficult to implement or does not exist.

One of the important implications of this regulatory guidance is the recognition of the utility of Bayesian methods in studies with relatively small populations, as is often the case with trials of medical devices. The EMEA has also noted the possible advantages of Bayesian methods in studies involving small populations[12]:

> Bayesian methods are a further source of 'adding assumptions' to data. They are a way to formally combine knowledge from previous data or prior 'beliefs' with data from a study. Such methods may be advantageous when faced with small datasets, although introducing

prior beliefs is often a concern in drug regulation. As with sensitivity analyses mentioned above, a variety of reasonable prior distributions should be used to combine with data from studies to ensure that conclusions are not too heavily weighted on the prior beliefs.

The advent of individualized medicine is likely to increase the number of studies for which only small populations of test subjects are available. As a result, the use of Bayesian methods may grow with the number of treatments that target populations based on genetic and other individual characteristics.

Conclusions

By allowing researchers to learn from data as it accumulates, the Bayesian approach opens new possibilities and provides new tools for clinical researchers. Bayesian methods have the advantage in early development of incorporating prior knowledge from a variety of sources, with strength of trial results overcoming different levels of skepticism about a drug's effects. Bayesian methods also allow greater flexibility in evaluating hypotheses, in interim monitoring, and in acting quickly when data justifies stopping trials early.

When Bayesian methods use uniform or noninformative priors, they have efficiency approximating that of frequentist studies and are likely to reach similar conclusions. However, reliance on prior distributions gives the Bayesian approach options that frequentist methods lack. These options include improving efficiency through informative prior distributions based on strong prior data, combining data on similar studies involving small populations when recruitment of larger populations is impossible, and starting with skeptical priors that reflect negative expert opinion or the belief that justification of a particular new drug requires extremely strong positive results. Bayesian methods also offer a straightforward way to analyze study results by using a variety of priors to gain a better understanding of the strength of evidence.

Frequentist methods have proved their value. However, their greatest strength lies in looking backward after studies conclude. There are frequentist methods for examining data at intervals, but each midcourse look calls for techniques to minimize the increase in error rates. As a result, frequentist methods seem fundamentally ill suited to incremental learning. Without a convenient mechanism for incremental learning, clinical research will have difficulty progressing toward the ideal of continuous development. There are times when the scientific method requires delays to ensure the soundness of learning. However, the need for some delays does not mean that all delays imposed by a specific methodology are good for science. Sometimes such delays reflect a weakness in methodology rather than a scientific virtue.

The capacity for incremental learning is inherent in the Bayesian approach. It is important to recognize that this capacity does not impose a requirement for intemperate haste. Bayesians, like frequentists, can pause to analyze data and consider next steps. However, the inherent capacity for incremental learning will sometimes allow studies and programs using Bayesian methods to acquire greater knowledge earlier. Together with strong support for interim decision making, the capacity for incremental learning will likely win greater acceptance for Bayesian methods over time.

Frequentists, Bayesians, and Pragmatists

Frequentist and Bayesian methods are not mutually exclusive approaches, and it is useful to consider each as providing tools that are sometimes complementary and sometimes better suited individually to certain tasks under different conditions. Statisticians increasingly see advantages in each approach, sometimes using the advantages of both approaches to address a single problem. Bayarri and Berger, for example, strongly urge the use of both approaches.[13] Little stresses the advent of tools that allow Bayesian methods to emerge as a practical alternative[14]:

> Whether or not the inferential debate has receded, it is no longer academic! Thirty years ago, applications of Bayes were limited to smallish problems by the inability to compute the high dimensional integrations involved in multiparameter models. Increased computational power and the development of Monte Carlo approaches to computing posterior distributions has turned this weakness of Bayes into a strength, and Bayesian approaches to large complicated models are now common in the statistical and scientific literatures.

Little finds today's statisticians divided into three main camps[14]:

(a) frequentists, who abhor the Bayesian approach or never learned much about it;

(b) Bayesians, with varying views on the role of frequentist ideas; and

(c) pragmatists, who do not have an overarching philosophy and pick and choose what seems to work for the problem at hand.

According to Little, pragmatists take the view that "good statisticians can get sensible answers under Bayes or frequentist paradigms; indeed maybe two philosophies are better than one, since they provide more tools for the statistician's toolkit!"[14] Little considers pragmatists in the ascendancy.

Adaptive studies can derive great benefit from the advent of Bayesian statistics as an alternative to the frequentist approach. On the other hand, the financial pressures and time constraints in the real world of drug development leave no alternative to pragmatism. With time, pragmatism will drive clinical researchers increasingly to choose the most appropriate frequentist or Bayesian tool for the immediate challenge. If necessary, biostatisticians will use a mixture of tools from both camps. When incremental learning or midcourse flexibility is essential for meeting development goals, Bayesian tools are likely to take a leading role.

Further information on Bayesian methods is available from a variety of sources.[15–22]

References

1 Salsburg D. The lady tasting tea. First Owl Books Edition. New York: Henry Holt and Company; 2002. pp. 111–2.

2 Neyman J, Pearson E. On the problem of the most efficient tests of statistical hypotheses. Philos Trans R Soc Ser A. 1933;231:289–337.

3 Dickens C. David Copperfield. 2000 Modern Library Paperback Edition. New York: Random House; 2000. p. 166.

4 Bayes T. An essay towards solving a problem in the doctrine of chances. (A Letter from the Late Reverend Mr. Thomas Bayes, F. R. S. to John Canton, M. A. and F. R. S.) Philos Trans R Soc. 1763;53:370–418.

5 Savage LJ. The foundations of statistics. Second revised edition. New York: Dover Publications, 1972.

6 Good IJ. A. M. Turing's statistical work in World War II. Biometrika. 1979;66:393–6.

7 Mosteller F, Wallace D. Applied Bayesian and classical inference: the case of the Federalist Papers. New York: Springer Verlag; 1984.

8 Fienberg S. When did Bayesian inference become "Bayesian"? Bayesian Anal. 2006;1:1–40.

9 Zdziarski J. Ending spam: Bayesian content filtering and the art of statistical language classification. San Francisco: No Starch Press; 2005.

10 U.S. Department of Health and Human Services, Food and Drug Administration, Center for Devices and Radiological Health. Guidance for the use of Bayesian statistics in medical device clinical trials—Draft guidance for industry and FDA staff . Washington (DC). May 2006. Available from: http://www.fda.gov/cdrh/osb/guidance/1601.html.

11 U.S. Department of Health and Human Services, Food and Drug Administration, Johns Hopkins University. Can Bayesian approaches to studying new treatments improve regulatory decision making. Bethesda (MD). May 20–21, 2004. Presentations available from: http://www.cfsan.fda.gov/~frf/bayesdl.html.

12 European Medicines Agency, Committee for Medicinal Products for Human Use. Guideline on clinical trials in small populations. London. July 2006. Available from: http://www.emea.europa.eu/pdfs/human/ewp/8356105en.pdf.

13 Bayarri MJ, Berger JO. The interplay of Bayesian and frequentist analysis. Statist Sci. 2004;19:58–80.

14 Little RJA. Calibrated Bayes: A Bayes/frequentist roadmap. Am Stat. 2006;60:213–23.

15 Austin PC, Brunner LJ, Hux JE. Bayeswatch: an overview of Bayesian statistics. J Eval Clin Pract. 2002;8:277–86.

16 Berry DA. Statistics: A Bayesian perspective. Pacific Grove, CA: Duxbury Press; 1995.

17 Spiegelhalter DJ, Abrams KR, Myles JP. Bayesian approaches to clinical trials and health-care evaluation. Chichester: John Wiley & Sons; 2004.

18 Berry DA. Bayesian statistics and the efficiency and ethics of clinical trials. Stat Sci. 2004;19:175–87.

19 Malakoff D. Bayes offers a 'new' way to make sense of numbers. Science. 1999;286:1460–4.

20 Berry D, Stangl D. Eds. Bayesian biostatistics. New York: Marcel Dekker; 1996.

21 Spiegelhalter DJ, Freedman SL, Parmar BKM. Bayesian approaches to randomized trials. J R Stat Soc (A). 1994;157:357–416.

22 Chow S, Chang M. Adaptive design methods in clinical trials. Boca Raton (FL): Chapman & Hall/CRC; 2007.

— Chapter 9 —

The Agile Platform

Before conducting adaptive studies or embracing agile clinical development, organizations should ensure that their technological infrastructure for clinical research can provide the timely information required. Typical infrastructure often fails to meet this test. Revisiting the Chapter 5 (page 120) example in which producing a seemingly simple screen failure report took several weeks and a substantial fee, it is clear that many CROs have limited ability to capture and process data rapidly and provide timely reports on even the most crucial data. Understanding the reasons for screen failures is essential for meeting timelines, and yet the necessary information is often unavailable. Study managers allow information to remain trapped on paper forms because no one recognizes the urgency of access to such information.

A contraceptive study that collected data with an interactive voice response system (IVRS) produced results inconsistent with those from a companion study that used paper diaries to collect the same data according to the same protocol. An investigation after the study revealed user frustration with the IVRS system as implemented. One subject complained, "The menus were confusing, and it was really hard to go back if you hit a wrong number. A lot of times, I ended up just not fixing errors or pushing any button to shut it up." Unaware of such user frustration and its effects, the study added data to the database without first examining it. When statisticians finally did look, they quickly realized that answers recorded for some patients made no sense. The variability exceeded the levels that study designers anticipated, as well as the variability in data collected by the companion study. Faced with the difficult choice between repeating the study and going to market with a product that reported much lower efficacy than they knew to be true, managers chose the latter.

A cycle of timely decision making drives agile research. The cycle works efficiently only if the technology platform can provide decision makers with the timely, accurate information they need when they need it. With each decision, the technology platform must also be capable of quickly communicating instructions to those responsible for implementation. Finally, the cycle must include the capability to track the effects of decisions, restarting the cycle.

Providing timely information for decision making requires three elements: capture of relevant data; validation and summary/analysis; and reporting appropriately for each individual's role. Because the goal is to enable timely decisions and actions, the presentation of information matters greatly. Clinical programs need information that serves the needs of sites, study management, and program management. Reports and presentations must distill mountains of raw data to meaningful summaries—frequencies, averages, distributions, changes from baseline, trends over time, and so on. The three-stage process of data capture, analysis, and reporting and presentation must operate continuously, accurately, and quickly. The process must also include the flexibility to change during a study or program to accommodate new or changed information needs.

Essential Types of Data

Agile research requires efficient capture of two general types of data: patient data and management data. Patient data consists of familiar trial measurements and observations. This includes the CRF data such as medical history, vital signs, laboratory results, X-rays, computerized tomography (CT) scans, electrocardiograms (EKGs), and so on, each as required by each study's goals. Many researchers assume patient data is the only data that matters in clinical studies. However, studies must have timely access to comprehensive management data in order to ensure the ability to obtain patient data.

There are two categories of management data, both essential. The first is performance metrics, measuring how well the study is performing key operations at any time. Examples of performance metrics include query rates, mean time to query response, and enrollment rate, both for the study as a whole and for individual sites. The second category of management data consists of performance analytics, which aid in understanding why performance metrics are good, bad, or indifferent. Performance analytics include reasons for screen failure, information about the effects of individual inclusion/exclusion criteria, a breakdown of enrollment by referral source, and information on which CRF fields generate more queries. Figure 9-1 summarizes the types of study data required for agile development.

Performance metrics identify areas that need improvement. Performance analytics suggest specific actions to correct shortcomings and increase efficiency in the areas identified.

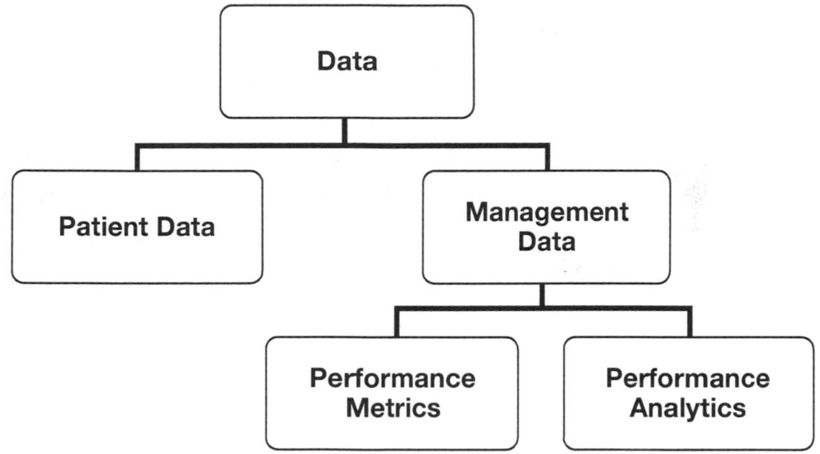

Figure 9-1. The types of study data required for agile clinical development.

All studies collect patient data. A minority collect performance metrics. Few studies collect and examine performance analytics. The agile platform must be capable of providing timely access not only to patient data but also to both types of management data—performance metrics and performance analytics.

Management Cycles in Clinical Studies

Both design adaptations and operational adaptations optimize clinical trials and programs through decision making based on timely, accurate information. The two types of adaptations involve processes that are the same at a general level but vary in practice.

Because the focus of design adaptations differs from that of operational adaptations, the two types often require different types of information, procedures, and decisions. Design adaptations rely on data from CRFs (Figure 9-2). Some design adaptations require data continuously; most require data at intervals. Response-adaptive randomization and adaptive dose finding often require continuous access to timely information. The former depends on timely outcome information as a basis for allocating each incoming patient to the appropriate treatment arm. Adaptive dose-finding techniques such as the CRM require timely information on patient response to decide on the appropriate dose for treating the next patient. Design adaptations that require data at intervals often time the intervals for scheduled review decisions, DSMB meetings, or milestones such as reaching half of the enrollment specified by planning estimates.

Even design adaptations that make a key decision or decisions at intervals can benefit from frequent access to timely data. For example, sample size reestimation during a study may not be time critical if the remaining planned enrollment extends months into the future. However, taking longer to clean data for the reestimation than it takes to enroll enough patients for the reestimation can undermine the entire exercise. Frequent measures of data quality allow earlier identification and cleanup of problems that might otherwise cause delays before episodic decisions. Leaving cleanup until the end can reduce time for analysis and deliberations, increase pressure on decision makers, and increase risk of poor judgments. For example, adaptive dose selection may involve decisions made at discrete intervals, but those decisions remain critically dependent on timely, accurate information for decisions to prune arms without causing delays or needlessly exposing additional patients to experimental treatments.

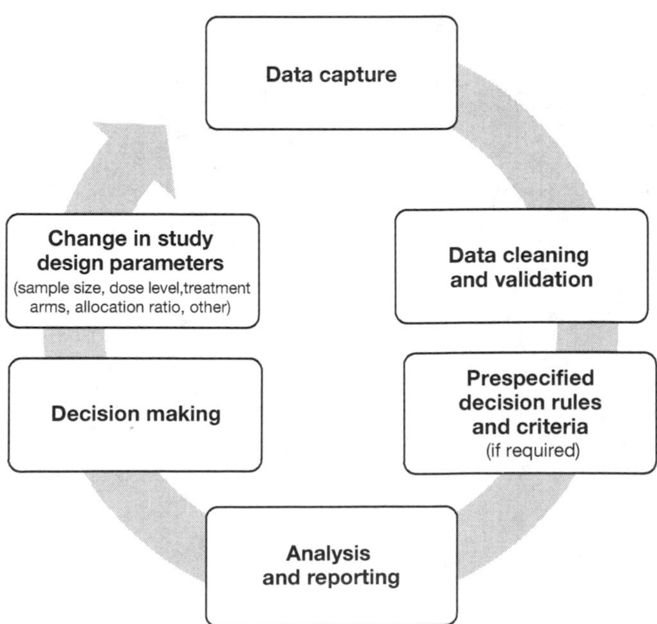

Figure 9-2. Management cycle for design adaptations.

The management cycle for operational adaptations focuses on performance metrics that track essential indicators of day-to-day study activities (Figure 9-3).

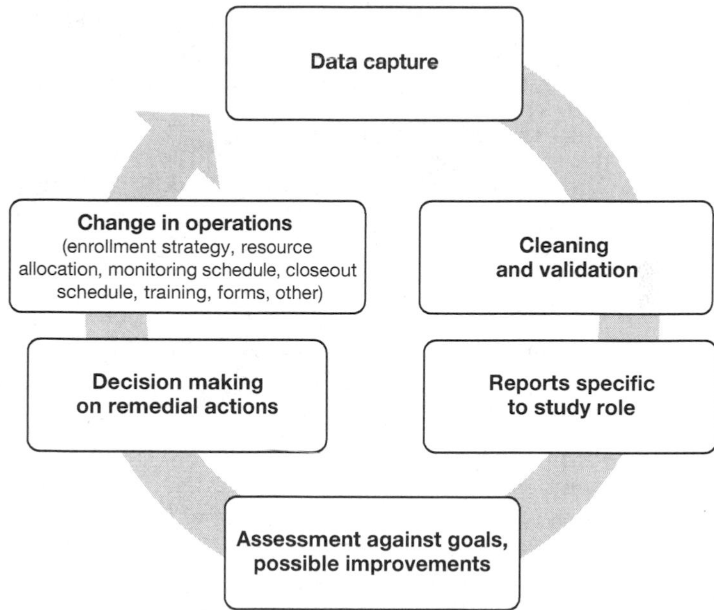
Data capture
Cleaning and validation
Reports specific to study role
Assessment against goals, possible improvements
Decision making on remedial actions
Change in operations
(enrollment strategy, resource allocation, monitoring schedule, closeout schedule, training, forms, other)

Figure 9-3. The management cycle for operational adaptations.

Because the goal of operational adaptations is to optimize day-to-day activities, decisions about operational adaptations always require capturing and analyzing a continuous stream of timely information. Otherwise, making and implementing decisions in time to manage a trial effectively becomes impossible. Adaptive enrollment relies on current information about the effectiveness of different recruitment techniques and the effects of specific inclusion/exclusion criteria. Adaptive monitoring allocates field resources based on quantity of data such as number of unmonitored fields and quality measures such as query rate, patterns in the nature of queries, and time to resolve queries. Adaptive site management requires current performance metrics on all major site activities. Timely site closeout and database lock become much easier if query resolution is prompt throughout a study, but prompt query resolution is essential toward the end.

Why Design Adaptations Are Dependent on Operational Adaptations

Ensuring the availability of current, accurate information for decisions on design adaptations requires efficient study operations up to that point. For example, delays in cleaning data and resolving queries can delay dose determination or randomization for the next incoming patient. Delays can put the undesired seam back into a study with a seamless design. Making design adaptations requires first applying the adaptive approach to the management of study operations. Otherwise, operational shortcomings can prevent the improvements in efficiency that motivated the use of design adaptations.

The Common Platform for Design and Operational Adaptations

The set of technologies needed to ensure timely availability of both data and performance metrics in clinical studies comprises the agile platform. The following pages explain the essential components and functions of this infrastructure. In some cases, the chapter will refer to necessary capabilities rather than specific products or technologies; in others, a technology or product already in use best illustrates necessary capabilities.

The central themes of the adaptive platform are rapid data collection and validation, the transformation of data into information to support decision making, and efficient study-wide communication of all data and information, but especially decisions intended to optimize the study. The remainder of this chapter examines components of the adaptive platform. The disproportionate attention to efficient data capture reflects an important reality. Without efficient data capture, the other components of the adaptive platform are moot. Conducting adaptive trials becomes impossible.

Data Capture

Rapid data capture is an essential starting point for effective research—but how rapid is rapid enough? The time between data capture on paper and availability in a study database once averaged six and one-half weeks because the norm was capturing data on paper and processing it in four-week batches. Today, in some trials using response-adaptive dose finding, data on the response of the most recently treated patient must be available almost immediately to allow selecting the dose for the next patient.

CONSIDERATIONS IN SELECTING A DATA CAPTURE APPROACH

How easy will sites find the method to use?

How well does the system mesh with site work patterns?

How hard is it to integrate the device with other systems?

How much training does the method require?

How accurate is the approach?

How long does it take to complete a CRF?

Are special skills required?

How many times is data transcribed?

In practice, achieving rapid data entry requires making the process of collecting and transmitting data as easy as possible for site personnel. Given human nature, any technology that makes data entry difficult or tedious will inevitably cause delays. The advantages of electronic data capture become an expensive illusion.

The choice of data-capture technologies should take into account the need for ready access not only to patient data but also to performance metrics for study management. The low direct costs of slow, paper-based systems seem less attractive in view of the inability of such systems to provide timely performance metrics. Similarly, EDC systems may fail to accelerate clinical studies if they slow down otherwise rapid electronic processes with rekeying of information and other transcription steps or if site personnel postpone data entry.

Selecting a data-capture technology also requires considering integration with clinical processes. Clinical data is an important output of some processes but an important input to others. Isolated measures to improve one component such as data capture may leave the processes with other bottlenecks that cancel the benefits. Technology's ability to improve the bottom line often requires defining a more efficient process and then applying technology in such a way as to improve performance of the process as a whole.

Data-Capture Technologies

Three generations of technologies compete in today's market for data-entry systems. The first generation consists of pen-and-paper data entry. The second generation includes faxback systems and web-based EDC, which both typically rely on paper data entry, require transcription steps, but then transmit data much more efficiently than first-generation systems. Another second-generation data-capture technology is IVRS systems. The third generation tries to improve efficiency by eliminating transcription steps. Third-generation systems include digital pens, tablet computers, and personal digital assistants (PDAs).

Each generation and each specific technology provide a different level of speed, accuracy, and ease of use. Ease of use affects both accuracy and speed of data availability, and so has enormous importance. Considerations that affect ease of use include the dimensions and clarity of data display, whether on standard paper, specialized forms, desktop computers, notebook computers, PDAs, or telephone handsets. The size and layout of keyboards and the number of available keys can make a big difference. When data input is by telephone, the standard keypad and absence of a display impose significant limitations. Input via PDA takes practice and skill because of small displays, specialized key layouts, and the need to learn the user interface for specific software used to collect and upload data. In addition, the fine motor skills for small devices may prove challenging for some groups.

The accompanying sidebar provides a checklist of additional considerations in evaluating data-capture technologies for clinical trials.

Despite the importance of ease of use for personnel at investigational sites, little information is available on comparative usability testing of data-capture methods for clinical trials. Many vendors for the market leading technology, web EDC, claim to perform usability testing and to offer superior usability. However, a search of current web EDC vendors found no publicly available comparative evaluations. One article urging usability testing of EDC systems notes, "EDC within the clinical trial environment presents a number of unique usability difficulties, including the physical location, the type of information collected, and personal characteristics of users; however, available EDC guidances only briefly mention usability."[1] The same article stresses the importance of validating the usability of any EDC system and understanding where it fits in workflow.

A few published studies shed some light on comparative ease of use of available data-capture technologies for clinical trials. In a study at an academic usability laboratory, the digital pen achieved highest marks for speed and accuracy of data capture, followed by keyboard data entry at a computer, the most common input method for EDC.[2] A PDA and tablet PC performed poorly by comparison. Digital pen and keyboard entry also received highest scores for ergonomics, mirroring scores on speed and accuracy.

An independent comparison of mobile data-capture technologies involving the digital pen, PDA, a hybrid PDA/digitizing tablet (a digitizing pad for input connected to a PDA for storage and communication), and a tablet PC found the digital pen the simplest to use. The pen generated fewest requests for technical help—8% of users, compared to 14% for tablet PC users, 42% for PDA/digitizing tablet, and 70% for PDA. Results indicated that the digital pen and the tablet PC surpassed other methods in ease of use and user satisfaction. Data capture with the digital pen also produced only about half as many errors as the combination of paper input followed by transcription.[3]

The First Generation

Pen and Paper

The first point of reference for data-capture methods is the time-honored paper CRF. Paper CRFs and forms are easy to use and inexpensive. However, they are also slow, labor intensive, and error prone. Site personnel normally transcribe data from source documents onto worksheets or CRFs, allow forms to accumulate, and then send batches of CRFs to a central location for keyboard input. The standard method for achieving high accuracy with paper forms is to have data-entry personnel enter every form twice. Thus, by design, half of the effort is redundant. The process associated with paper data often takes a month or more between data generation and electronic entry and validation. Site personnel often receive faxed queries and submit corrections to a centralized database monitor. Because data remains unavailable in electronic form for such long periods, data capture by paper forms is wholly inadequate for adaptive trials.

The Second Generation

Web-Based Electronic Data Capture

The leading candidate to replace paper data capture is web-based EDC. Web-based EDC systems shift keyboard entry to local sites, offering site personnel immediate but limited feedback, such as range checks. Expectations for the benefits of web-based EDC were once high. Many observers consider results in the field disappointing:

> Electronic data capture (EDC) systems became available in the marketplace with the expectation that efficiencies gained in other web-based markets would now be brought to clinical data capture. To date, many would agree that such efficiencies are still not apparent,

> mainly due to the continued use of processes involving paper-based data collection.[4]

A 2007 estimate suggested that one-half of clinical studies initiated would be using EDC by the end of that year.[5] Penetrating only half the market by such a late date seems a limited accomplishment when the competition is paper. To investigational sites, web-based EDC systems have been at best a mixed blessing. Medical professionals at the sites take on the unwelcome chore of data entry. Sponsors have also imposed a variety of data-capture programs with inconsistent user interfaces, often on dedicated notebook computers for each study. Separate computers simplify maintaining confidentiality of study data. However, sponsors have at times acknowledged site complaints about having to use as many as five different notebook computers simultaneously for different studies.[6]

Some pharma companies also have reservations about transferring the task of data entry to investigational sites. The head of data management at a large pharmaceutical company told the author: "I'm just transferring data entry from my shop, where I control what happens, to the field, where I don't. The speed of data entry and availability of data have been a big disappointment, and overall, there has been little improvement in timelines or cost."

In practice, web-based EDC systems still initiate data capture with paper input, whether because of the desire for a paper copy of original input or because sites prefer to collect original patient data on paper rather than at a keyboard during a patient visit. Most EDC systems require multiple transcriptions steps. After abstracting information from the source document to an intermediate worksheet, site personnel keyboard data from the worksheet into an online system. During keyboard entry, the system transmits data to a central point, where automated procedures check each point against a predefined acceptable range. Systems typically perform consistency checks after large batches of data accumulate. Nevertheless, web-based EDC systems can pass through or introduce errors that fall within acceptable ranges and therefore evade error checks.

Disappointing results from web-based EDC have as much to do with where they fit in the larger processes of clinical research as with inherent limitations:

> The reviews of EDC are mixed to date, but few believe EDC has provided the efficiency gains expected when it began. One of the important reasons for this lack of success is the lack of commitment to process change required to achieve the sizable benefits industry believes are possible. Process change requires looking at the complete process and improving it, not simply continuing an inefficient process in a web-based approach. The reality is that the process of

> collecting clinical data is essentially the same as it was through the 1970s when data was computerized centrally and continuing through the 1980s and 1990s using RDE (Remote Data Entry) and now using EDC. Efficiency gains are possible in EDC when we look to identify the inefficient processes in current EDC and work to improve them in conjunction with the use of the internet.[4]

Debate remains about the extent to which real web-based EDC systems actually improve data capture, cleaning, and delivery. If site personnel enter data earlier, EDC certainly makes data available sooner in electronic form. Web-based EDC has also accelerated data checks by comparison with awaiting a CRA visit.

Few people praise web-based EDC for its ease of use. The sites that do the keyboarding generally often believe web-based EDC increases their workload. The process at the center is manually keyboarding data, which is notoriously prone to error. In EDC's favor, the input technology is the standard PC that millions of people use every day. On the other hand, many people still find PC user interfaces confusing. This problem is common when using different applications to perform similar work, as is the case for site personnel using different EDC systems for different studies.

Any significant delay between the generation of data at a site and the availability of the data to guide decision makers undermines the adaptive approach. One company active in adaptive trials advises companies that existing EDC systems may not be up to the task. The company recommends using a second, parallel EDC system, "EDC Lite," to ensure adequate performance "if the main EDC cannot produce response data quickly, frequently and reliably."[7] Having to recommend installing a second EDC system to conduct an adaptive trial speaks to the suitability of common EDC systems for adaptive trials.

Faxback Systems

Faxback systems have enjoyed a resurgence following significant recent improvements. Fax machines and fax features in computer systems are in every office. Faxing is generally easy despite the occasional busy signal, dropped call, or paper feed issue. Technological advances have minimized the old drawbacks of dealing with data in image form and tying up telephone lines. Early faxback systems involved faxing in forms to an office where people read the forms and keyed in data manually. However, recent versions incorporate optical mark and character recognition technology to read the incoming forms with impressive accuracy. This capability improves on the rekeying process of web-based EDC. It also makes it easy to manage data at a centralized location with a dedicated staff. Unlike web-based EDC, tablet PCs, and PDAs, faxback systems are not interactive. Nevertheless, recent improvements have extended the life of the fax as a data-capture technology for clinical trials. Appropriately implemented with machine-readable input, this system can be configured to provide data quickly enough to allow use for the most demanding aspect of adaptive studies, adaptive randomization.

Interactive Voice Response Systems

Interactive voice response systems are telephone-based systems that record data entered on a telephone keypad or spoken through a handset. IVRSs have proved useful for certain types of information such as patient responses and diaries. Suitable applications typically have relatively few questions and collect unambiguous information such as integers on a numeric response scale. IVRSs have the advantage of a familiar user interface that virtually everybody can use. On the other hand, users may require a paper form to guide them through the voice-input process, and the interactive dialogue may consume more of the user's time than filling out a paper form. Although IVRSs can perform range checks, the process increases the time required for input, possibly straining the patience of the person on the telephone. This presents a dilemma when ensuring the receipt of reasonable data requires range checks.[8]

IVRSs are not appropriate for standard data collection during a trial if, as is often the case, data collection involves many pages, branching and optional questions, and other complexities too demanding for input via a telephone handset. Whether an IVRS is appropriate for adaptive research depends on the complexity of the data required by each study.

The Third Generation

The Digital Pen

The digital pen captures data in electronic form and yet does not require the ability to operate a computer. It is easy to carry, has a long battery life, and allows keeping a paper record without carrying along a computer and a printer. Several vendors provide digital pen hardware and software for creating paper forms for data collection, including Logitech, Hewlett-Packard, and Anoto. One company is conducting numerous clinical trials using 1,400 digital pens,[9] citing investigators' distaste for acting as EDC data-entry clerks and the distraction of typing on computer keyboards during patient visits.[10] Other companies have used the digital pen in trials with as many as 4,000 patients; one recently launched study using the digital pen includes 10,000 patients (Richard Farris, Health Decisions, personal communications).

All the comparative studies cited at the beginning of the data-capture section look favorably on the digital pen. Another independent study of data-capture technology assessed the use of a digital pen in a clinical trial.[11] A Hewlett-Packard digital pen performed data capture in an ongoing sequential trial that compared two antiplatelet therapy strategies. To analyze data accuracy, the investigators arranged for keyboard double data entry of printouts of the forms showing handwritten input. The study found no significant difference in accuracy between double entry and pen entry. Some digital pen users expressed the wish for instantaneous data availability. Two trial participants familiar with EDC systems preferred the digital pen. One commented:

> It's much quicker than Internet data entry. I've used internet data entry and found it to be tedious, time-consuming, and generally terrible. But the pen is easy, it's like a normal pen, you fill in a form just as you would normally do then you are done. It's great, really.[11]

Digital pen users write the same way as with a conventional pen but on special paper that has a fine dot pattern that appears as a pale background on the printed sheet. The dots enable the pen to recognize the form and locations on the form through a camera in the pen's tip. As the clinician writes, the pen stores each pen stroke in an internal nonvolatile memory. Following completion of a form or forms, the pen may communicate over a wireless network (Bluetooth), through a wireless telephone, or through a dock attached to a PC.[9] The intermediary device transmits data to a central location, sometimes immediately. The central location translates each keystroke to checks, numbers, and letters using a combination of optical mark and character recognition. Depending on the implementation, software may perform automated data validation immediately. The accuracy of such data-capture systems far surpasses keyboard entry of data (~96–99% accuracy) by achieving 99.96% accuracy, depending on the receiving software and systems. In the previously cited French study, accuracy was 99.8% when transmission failures are included and 99.9% when they are not.[11] Even if the pen simultaneously records data with ink on paper, the data originates in electronic form, allowing immediate transmission to the study database. Pen hardware and a paper form create an electronic record; printable images correspond exactly but the original record is usually electronic.

Uploading data by docking the pen after a patient visit can make data available even before a patient leaves the site. Study staff can also send queries almost immediately. This provides a quick opportunity not only to correct erroneous data but also to alert site personnel to a problem with the data entered in order to prevent recurrences of avoidable input problems. Following this approach produces clean data much more quickly and decreases the query rate below that of any of the other data-capture systems discussed here. The electronic pen CRF can also serve as source material (i.e., the first recording of a value), obviating the need to send monitors to the site to do source verification of electronic data against paper forms. The digital pen meets the demands of adaptive trials for timely, accurate data for management.

The Tablet PC

Tablet PCs allow pen input with a stylus on a touch-sensitive screen (Figure 9-4). These specialized PCs can display the equivalent of a full paper CRF. Like PDAs, tablet PCs allow interaction with an onboard computer and through wireless communications. However, tablet PCs cost more than PDAs or typical notebook computers. In the current generation, tablet PCs remain too bulky and heavy for most medical professionals to consider for routine use recording data on patient visits. Furthermore, multiple studies with their own dedicated tablet PCs or notebook computers complicate work at investigational sites. The portability of the tablet PC loses some of its appeal with the inconvenience of carrying several computers from room to room or fetching a different computer before examining each patient. A variety of other data-capture systems, including web-based EDC and the digital pen, can run the same software as tablet PCs.

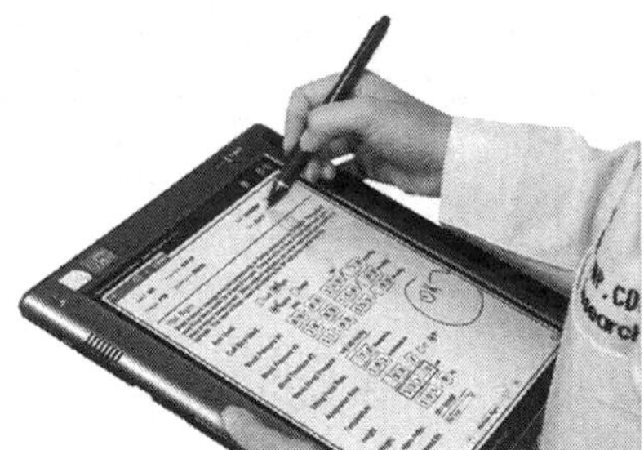

Figure 9-4. Tablet PC for data capture, which immediately converts input to text.

As computers become lighter and smaller, purpose-built machines will facilitate specific applications in hospitals and clinical settings. Electronic medical records also promise a common entry system someday that might encourage use of purpose-built devices. However, issues such as validation for research, patient confidentiality and integration present formidable obstacles to widespread adoption of electronic medical records in the immediate future. As technology evolves, tablet PCs or their descendants may ultimately provide the best balance of convenience, portability, and flexibility for data capture in clinical trials.

PDAs and Handheld Computers

The small devices known as PDAs or handheld computers (HHCs) provide a combination of easy transportability and full interactivity. This combination seems attractive for applications such as capturing data on patient visits. However, pocket-sized portable computers compromise usability and thus complicate recording clinical data. These compact devices have small, nonstandard keypads. They also have screens much smaller and more difficult to read than typical case report forms. Some reports do comment favorably on the use of PDAs in clinical studies, especially in studies where portability is at a premium, such as in remote settings.[12] Another successful use of PDAs has been in patient diaries that allow inputting self-assessments of response to treatment.[13]

On the other hand, a clinical trial that used handheld computers for a subset of patients suggested notable limitations in data capture by PDAs. The trial entered data on a subset of patients using both paper forms and the handheld PCs. The error rate for data captured with the handheld computers was 67.[14] per 10,000 fields compared to the "accepted" rate of 10 errors per 10,000 fields for double data entry from paper forms. Users reported discomfort using the handheld devices for data entry. They also complained about technical problems uploading data.[14] Technology improves over time, but the handheld computer's size seems a long-term handicap for capturing patient data in clinical trials.

PDAs have secured a place in health care by providing portable data access, scheduling, and reference. These devices also do a good job of capturing patient diaries on simple CRFs.[15]

Comparative Strengths and Weaknesses

Table 9-1 summarizes the benefits and limitations of the most competitive data-capture technologies. Since telephone voice-response systems, IVRSs and PDAs have proved less suitable for capturing the large volume of CRF data, this table omits these technologies. The table draws on direct experience with several data-capture technologies, the author's analysis of data-capture processes, interaction with site staff for numerous studies, and the articles cited earlier. As such, the table is a mixture of objective information and personal observation summarizing benefits and limitations. The table does not purport to be a rigorous scientific comparison of the technologies.

Table 9-1. Comparative performance, cost, and suitability of methods for capturing CRF data for adaptive studies.

Method	Benefits	Limitations	Number of Transcription Steps
Paper	Simple, intuitive	Slow	1
Web-based EDC	Limited concurrent validation	Requires keyborad entry; increases site work; training and support; integration with other systems	2–3
Faxback	Simple, intuitive; no keyboard entry; minimal training	Can be time consuming	1
Digital pen	Simple, intuitive electronic entry; web or phone		0–1
Tablet PC	Quick, intuitive	Initial expense, support; extensive programming	0–1

Figure 9-5 compares two key measures of data-capture performance for five technologies.

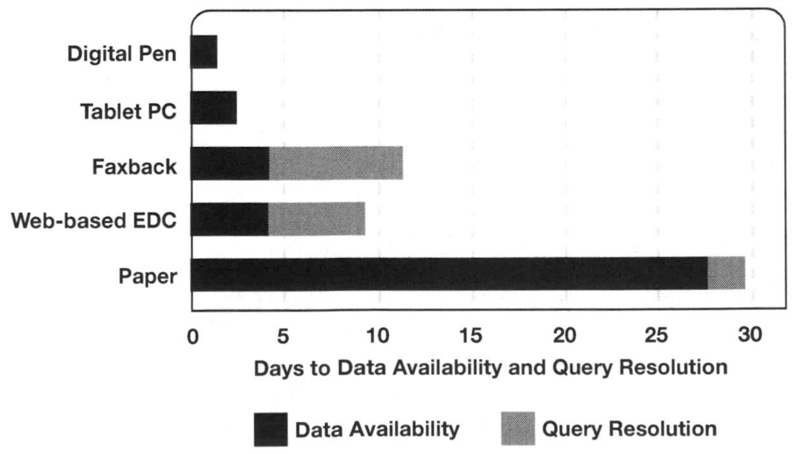

Figure 9-5. Typical time to clean data for different data-collection methods. This involves both initial collection of data and resolution of associated queries.

Table 9-1. Continued across from previous page.

Accuracy (Query Rate/100 fields)	Direct Cost	Time to Data Availability	Suitability for Adaptive Research
12-35	$	Weeks	—
7-9	$$$$	Days	✓
3-10	$$	Hours	✓✓
0.5-1	$$	Minutes	✓✓✓
Insufficient data	$$$$	Minutes	✓✓✓

Data Cleaning and Validation Technology

Data acquisition is the first step toward getting usable data quickly. However, this step in isolation is of no practical use. The subsequent steps of validation and cleaning, summarization, and reporting make data useful. This entire process must perform at a high level in fast-moving adaptive programs. Decision making in adaptive research depends not only on capturing data but also on assuring accuracy. Inaccuracy or slowness to assure accuracy becomes the rate-limiting step for adaptive decisions.

Data validation involves range checks, consistency checks, and trend checks. Range checks determine that a value falls within specified limits. Consistency checks determine whether data on different portions of a questionnaire agree when necessary. For example, data should not indicate that the same subject is both male and pregnant. Trend checks identify surprising changes over time. Laboratory values over several visits may all fall within range limits, and yet the sudden appearance of a value at the bottom of the range deserves scrutiny if preceding values have all been near the top. Range, consistency, and trend checks may be independent of one another. All require careful evaluation. In practice, studies usually focus on range checks to the neglect of checks for consistency and trends.

Some types of errors are difficult to detect. Of particular note are erroneous values within allowable limits but nonetheless incorrect. Such errors are more common when data capture requires reentry of data by people who lack training to increase keyboarding accuracy.

Some recent systems perform more sophisticated data checks. A trend of declining values over time, even within range limits, may serve as an early warning of safety or other problems. In a study of hemodialysis patients, an advanced validation system detected an otherwise overlooked pattern of subtle decreases in hemoglobin levels. Systems incorporating neural networks can sometimes spot trends early and rapidly identify the types of errors that occur at a given site or by a given interviewer. Such systems not only detect errors but also seek to identify and correct the underlying causes. Errors often indicate more than just a discrepancy between expected and actual values. Managers should assume that each error indicates a problem that can waste time and resources. On this assumption, the correct response to each query includes uncovering information essential for achieving greater efficiency.

A bottom-line measure of good data capture is the query rate, which also indicates the amount of rework required to ensure correct data.

Data Analysis Tools

Decision making in adaptive trials requires continuous review of incoming data and performance metrics, whether adaptations involve study design or operations. Decisions about dose escalation, dynamic patient allocation, and treatment pruning often require rapid access to reliable information. For some adaptive methods, such as rising dose-escalation studies, rapid data access can cut the phase time by 80% or more (see Chapter 6). Operational adaptations demand the same immediacy to prevent repetitive errors from proliferating on a scale that undermines the efficiency of key trial processes and the study as a whole.

Design and operational adaptations both demand a combination of automated checking and human review of certain types of data. The goal is to flag exceptions not only to specified ranges but also to historical and expected patterns and trends. Although most web-based EDC systems provide immediate feedback to keyboard data entry at a PC, the supporting systems lack the capacity to detect and analyze complex patterns.

Data analysis rests on the ability to execute straightforward checks such as range checks quickly and the ability to analyze and learn from complex patterns. Current industry practice addresses the former with care but offers at best limited capabilities for addressing the latter. Apart from simple range checks, consistency and other checks flag fields for review by data specialists. A single error in answers to related questions can trigger multiple queries. Sites find it frustrating when one simple error produces a flurry of queries.

Improving data analysis requires greater reliance on automation, including systems that can address more of the complexities that currently require human intervention. Automated systems must also improve the ability to trace problems to their origin. For example, a certain group of sites, an individual site, or an individual interviewer may have a persistent problem. The goal of the data-processing system must be both to speed the process of validation through maximum use of automation and to shorten the feedback loop by issuing error notices faster, such as queries and notices to sites about likely causes of errors.

Randomization

Randomization, integral to many adaptive designs, requires immediate, clean data for rapid decision making. Randomization that depends on continuous responses to differing doses or continuous tracking of covariates requires automated collection, assessment, and reporting. Some randomization schemes are complex. For example, some require examining not only responses to a given dose but also responses to adjacent doses. Such schemes demand rapid accuracy checks and rapid reports in formats that facilitate decision making.

The common failure to crosscheck data derived from patient information poses risks for adaptive randomization. Many different issues can undermine accuracy. For example, elderly users may lack dexterity to hit telephone response buttons, producing errors that are random (keys around the intended key) or systematic (above or below the intended key, depending on motor capabilities). If there is no other means of checking entered data, no written record, then there is no way of assessing the accuracy of the data. The validation built into randomization systems should always include commonsense checks to ensure that patients are both eligible and appropriate, since many intention-to-treat analyses will include every patient randomized. Checks should also include trends for individuals and outliers for any value.

Studies rely increasingly on centralized randomization to ensure precise control. Centralized randomization allows halting randomization studywide as soon as the study meets enrollment goals. Randomization systems must be able to address issues such as stratification according to factors that affect outcome measures, such as disease severity. Furthermore, randomization systems should be capable of ensuring even distribution of factors such as demographic characteristics among treatment groups to limit the possible influence of unknown or unmeasurable risk factors. Finally, such a system must be able to support different types of randomization, including response-adaptive and multivariate-adaptive randomization.

Site Management

Although site performance does much to determine study performance, studies typically do little to help sites perform their tasks more efficiently. Often the cause of such neglect is the failure of infrastructure to provide information essential for rapid identification of site issues and diagnosis of causes. Optimizing site performance requires infrastructure that continuously tracks and measures performance of key tasks for the study as a whole and all sites individually. Because handling a needlessly heavy volume of queries compromises site performance, one of the most important capabilities for infrastructure is continuously tracking queries and query resolution. The focus should be on minimizing queries, not just addressing queries one at a time.

Controlling the number of queries requires developing an early understanding of why queries are occurring. To this end, it is important to have technology that provides performance analytics such as a breakdown of query rates by CRF question, by site, and by interviewer. Figure 9-6 illustrates a system that helps managers analyze the performance by site.

Site ID	Subjects Involved	Total Pages	Queries Generated	Computer Queries	Manual Queries	Queries Released	Outstanding Queries	Overdue Queries	Pages Per Query
2	276	8312	1090	959	131	548	19	0	7.6
Overall	216	8312	1090	959	131	548	19	0	7.6

			Generated Queries				Released Queries			
Subjects Involved	Total Pages	Database Fields	Queries Generated	Pages Per Query	Queries Per Subject	Fields Per Query	Queries Released	Pages Per Query	Queries Per Subject	Fields Per Query
216	8312	23239	1090	7.6	5.0	21.3	548	15.2	2.5	42.4

Figure 9-6. Information that helps managers analyze query patterns at individual sites. The data shown provides insight into queries at a single site. Study infrastructure must generate such metrics continuously to meet the performance standards of adaptive studies and agile development.

Supply-Chain Management

Adaptive studies move fast and demand rapid, flexible supply-chain management to achieve objectives such as reducing timelines and costs. In studies with rapidly changing allocation, the supply chain can delay patient treatment and data collection, frustrating adaptive goals. Study infrastructure plays a key role in ensuring that the supply chain meets the requirements of adaptive methods. One requirement is a CTMS that can track drug supplies for each site according to criteria that may change with each iteration of an adaptive process. Suppose a trial at first gives each site a two-week supply of drugs reflecting initial estimates of promising doses. When the study randomizes a patient to an arm with a certain dose, a central system would decrement the supply of that dose. When supplies fall below a prespecified level based on maintaining a two-week buffer, resupply occurs automatically, with an e-mail to the site and the monitor responsible for the site. Each site maintains a projected duration of supply that preserves the buffer. For example, if all sites initially receive an estimated two-week supply and one site enrolls so slowly that the supply will last for four weeks, the study can reallocate the excess for the slow site to a faster-enrolling site with greater needs.

Adaptive randomization changes the background supply requirements. If an initial allocation ratio of 1:1:1 for three doses gradually shifts to 3:2:1, drug ordering and distribution shifts accordingly. Toward the end of the study, the study can gradually reduce the buffer supply. When a dosing arm or site completes the treatment cycle, then the study can ship any remaining drug to other sites.

A centralized CTMS should be capable of forecasting and managing complex supply needs. Some studies must be able to state where each individual drug sample is at any time. To address such needs, an integrated CTMS should incorporate a tracking system that records each instance of a study drug, CRF binder, or any study supply throughout the study. The system should track usage at each site, project needs, replenish automatically, and allow supplies to be shifted from one site to another. Needs will always differ from one site to another, and the amount of buffer built in will differ as well. Drugs or devices that are expensive will require closer just-in-time management. Meeting the needs of some studies requires geographic resupply centers. Supply management must be able to treat all the sites in the U.S. separately from all the sites in Europe. In supply-chain management for adaptive studies, the watchwords are precision, flexibility, and timeliness.

Communications

Communications provide the vital link between managers and the people and sites they manage and between individuals and the information they need to do their jobs. The final requirement for agile development is a rapid, effective means of transmitting information to individuals performing and managing studies and programs.

The web is the simplest technology for efficient, around-the-clock communications on a global scale. A custom study website can provide:

- Immediate, study-wide communication without regard to geography.
- Constant, universal access to necessary study documents, ranging from protocols to protocol amendments to forms (1572s, etc).
- Immediate feedback about performance relative to other sites. This is critical for some functions (competitive enrollment) and desirable for others. Peer pressure is a powerful motivator.
- A mechanism for instant communication of site issues and concerns to study management.
- Ready access to hard figures for incentives and disincentives. If a study can drop sites for poor performance, the sites must understand the performance metrics.

Conclusions

Realizing the benefits of adaptive methods and the agile approach to clinical development requires infrastructure that can perform at a high level. Notoriously poor performance versus research timelines and budgets reflects the inadequacy of a typical infrastructure. When the infrastructure is incapable of keeping study managers current on the status of operations or providing the timely information required for decisions about design adaptations, improving the efficiency of clinical research is a pipe dream. A capable infrastructure, the agile platform, provides the foundation for techniques that can lift efficiency to unprecedented heights.

References

1 Schmier JK, Kane DW, Halpern MT. Practical applications of usability theory to electronic data collection for clinical trials. Contemp Clin Trials. 2005;26:376–85.

2 Boldt R, Raasch J. Analysis of current technologies and devices for mobile data capture: A qualitative usability-study for comparison of data capture via keyboard, tablet PC, personal digital assistant, and digital pen and paper. Usability lab of the department of computer science at the Hochschule für Angewandte Wissenschaften. Oct 2, 2008.

3 Cole E, Pisano ED, Clary GJ, Zeng D, Koomen M, Kuzmiak CM, Seo BK, Lee Y, Pavic D. A comparative study of mobile electronic data entry systems for clinical trials data collection. Int J Med Inform. 2006;75:722–9.

4 Marks RG. Validating electronic source data in clinical trials. Controlled Clin Trials. 2004;25:437–46.

5 Connor C. U.S. electronic data capture 2006–2011: Spending forecast and analysis. Health Industry Insights. Apr 30, 2007.

6 Senior M. Making clinical trials more efficient. In Vivo: The Business and Medicine Report. 2005;23:1–6.

7 Parke T. Adaptive clinical trials in the real world. Presentation to the Massachusetts Biotechnology Council. Apr 23, 2008. Slide 29, EDC lite. Available from: www.massbio.org/writable/committees/presentations/mbc__act_in_the_real_world.ppt; cited Dec, 11 2008.

8 Abu-Hasaballah K, James A, Aseltine RH Jr. Lessons and pitfalls of interactive voice response in medical research. Contemp Clin Trials. 2007;28:593–602.

9 Fröderberg U. Pen power. Int Clin Trials. 2008;3:32–8.

10 Borfitz D. Actelion opts for digital pen and paper over EDC. BioITWorld eCliniqua. Oct 1, 2007. Available from: http://www.bio-itworld.com/newsitems/2007/oct/01-digital-pen-and-paper/; cited Dec 11, 2008.

11 Estellat C, Tubach F, Costa Y, Hoffmann I, Mantz J, Ravaud P. Data capture by digital pen in clinical trials: A qualitative and quantitative study. Contemp Clin Trials. 2008;29:314–23.

12 Missinou MA, et al. Short report: Piloting paperless data entry for clinical research in Africa. Am J Trop Med Hyg. 2005;72:301–3.

13 Lane SJ, Heddle NM, Arnold E, Walker I. A review of randomized controlled trials comparing the effectiveness of hand held computers with paper methods for data collection. BMC Medical Informatics and Decision Making. 2006;6:23.

14 Shelby-James T, Abernethy A, McAlindon A, Currow DC. Handheld computers for data entry: high tech has its problems too. Trials. 2007;8:5.

15 Matthew AG, et al. Personal digital assistant data capture: The future of quality of life measurement in prostate cancer treatment. J Oncol Pract. 2007;3:115–20.

— Chapter 10 —

The Future of Clinical Development

This book describes an approach to clinical development that promises far greater efficiency. Because clinical testing comprises a high proportion of development costs and timelines, this more efficient approach would allow the pharma industry to take drugs from discovery to regulatory approval much faster and at lower cost. Seizing this opportunity requires systematic changes like those that other industries have used to achieve what the pharma industry needs now: a leap in efficiency. Tentative, incremental changes in a decades-old approach to clinical research will not produce such a leap. Only decisive action will do.

The need for dramatic improvements in clinical development is beyond debate. The combination of higher costs and declining output of new drugs has placed the pharma industry under unsustainable financial strain. In the midst of such financial pressures, the industry faces demands to meet several new challenges. These include better protecting test subjects and patients who receive new treatments, developing therapies for maladies afflicting small patient populations, and realizing the promise of individualized therapies. The high cost of the current approach to clinical development makes it all but impossible to meet such demands. The industry can address its financial pressures and other demands only through greater efficiency.

The action required to improve efficiency is to take full advantage of the great advances in communications and computing in the decades since the introduction of the approach that still dominates clinical research. Adaptive research provides the means of taking this bold step forward. The required changes must be extensive and systematic. However, the move to adaptive methods does not require large capital investments, new science, technological breakthroughs, or compromises in scientific standards. The path to greater efficiency consists almost entirely of techniques proven in other industries and, to a limited degree, in clinical research as well.

Adaptive research amounts to allowing common sense to play a greater role in clinical studies. In daily life, almost everyone makes frequent changes in response to new information. The few people who maintain course without considering new information meet Einstein's definition of insanity: "Doing the same thing over and over again and expecting different results." Common sense says that getting different results requires doing things differently. The black-box approach of running long, expensive trials to completion based on initial guesses made sense in an era when technology was incapable of providing midcourse information. Today, this approach is as anachronistic as an abacus. Moreover, the prevailing approach has in recent years produced miserable results. Openness to new processes and tools will allow the industry to discover an attractive, pragmatic alternative to doing the same thing over and over again and hoping for different results—making the same huge investments in clinical development only to see the same disappointing output of new drugs every year.

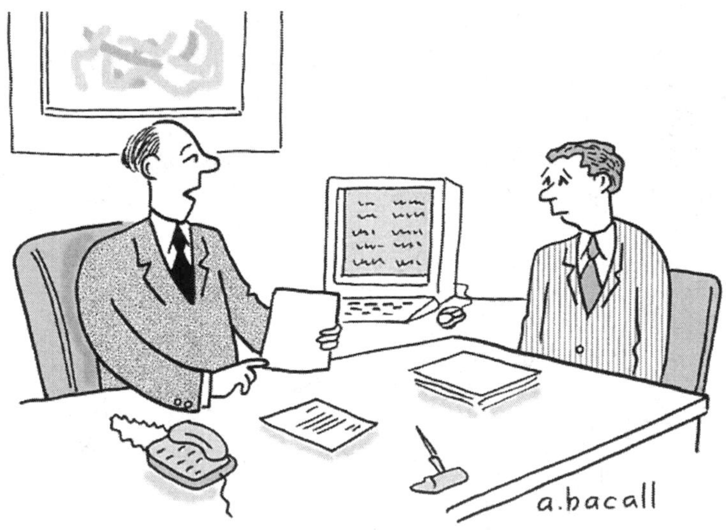

"This really is an innovative approach, but I'm afraid we can't consider it. It's never been done before."

What allows the injection of more common sense into clinical studies is the advent of adaptive methods. Such methods do not supplant scientific judgment and experimental design. Rather, adaptive methods supplement these essentials while also allowing more effective study management. Simply put, adaptive methods allow changing both study design and study operations in response to new information. In contrast to rigid designs that test a single hypothesis without considering data collected during a trial, adaptive studies can shift in response to new data, with each new piece of information contributing to the direction from that point forward. Adaptive methods acknowledge the uncertainty inherent in scientific research and provide a pragmatic response. Like the prevailing approach to study design, the current approach to study operations makes plans based on initial guesses and follows plans without change. The lack of meaningful, timely information on the status of key activities such as enrollment, monitoring, and site closeout leaves study managers no basis for adjusting strategy and procedures.

Adaptive methodologies provide the ability to make changes as necessary to reduce waste, shorten timelines, acquire superior information about drug candidates, and make the most productive use of development funds. The ability to adapt study designs can identify the least and most promising drug candidates earlier, improve the selection of doses for late-stage trials, and bring successful candidates to market faster. Adapting study operations based on real-time data and performance metrics promises even greater improvements in the efficiency of drug development. Optimizing key operations such as enrollment, site monitoring, and site closeout can prevent common delays, eliminate waste, and reduce costs. Finally, a comprehensive approach—agile clinical development—leverages information technology and optimizes processes for adapting both study designs and operations, maximizing efficiency in individual clinical studies and entire development programs.

This chapter summarizes how adaptive methods and agile clinical development can allow the industry to surmount its growing challenges. However, for observers who believe restructuring and consolidation can assure the industry a brighter future, I will first explore whether these measures really provide an alternative strategy for addressing the industry's problems. Then, taking the industry's challenges one at a time, the chapter will show how improvements in clinical development can allow the industry to respond effectively and secure its future despite trying circumstances.

Is Restructuring an Alternative to Improving Clinical Development?

The most pressing question for the drug industry is not whether it faces an urgent need for change. It does. For the present, the industry can still decide the nature of that change. On the one hand, the industry can initiate changes typical of maturing industries—successive waves of head-count reductions, consolidation, and growing aversion to risk as reflected in an effort to maintain current profits by cutting expenditures, such as R&D, that are not expected to provide near-term revenues and profits. Industry leaders may see the future as a contest to be among the few who survive in the equivalent of the car industry's Big Three. The handful of survivors would measure success in terms of maintaining profits by increasing share in a mature market. However, surviving one wave of contraction in such a market does not guarantee surviving the next. Detroit again provides an example. The once unassailable Big Three may dwindle to a Big Two, with one of the two in bankruptcy.

Other industries have faced similar decisions about their future direction at similar crossroads. For half a century, the American car industry has failed to confront the need to make better products more efficiently. Meanwhile, Japanese companies have achieved preeminence by developing systematic techniques for consistently producing superior automobiles faster and at lower cost. Toyota's innovative thinking about development and production resulted in more efficient processes based on continuous improvement and ruthless elimination of everything that hampered the ability to produce products to meet market needs. Toyota took a fresh look at supposedly optimal methods of mass production perfected by dominant American firms, found major inefficiencies, and swept them aside. In 2008, Toyota eclipsed General Motors as the world's largest car company. Toyota has succeeded not through dramatic changes but through optimized processes for consistently and continuously improving how the company works. Spasmodic American efforts to catch up have proved no match for a system that institutionalizes continuous improvement.

Many companies in a variety of industries have drawn on lessons from Toyota's success to achieve much greater efficiency. Manufacturing, an area where competition keeps margins low, was among the first industries to embrace Toyota's lean methods and to employ information technology to provide superior management based on a continuous flow of real-time information. The steel industry in the United States underwent a painful transition with slow, capital-intensive behemoths giving way to vigorous small competitors that used new management methods and flexible minimills.

Reductions in military subsidies drove the aerospace industry to embrace lean principles, with impressive results. For example, the preparation of a kit of materials and tools needed for a particular task reduced the time required to apply tape to B-2 bombers from 8.4 to 1.6 hours. A factory that manufactures fan cowls, part of the nacelle surrounding the engine for the Boeing 717, replaced a process that had moved metal 17,000 feet in 43 days with an approach that achieved the same result by moving metal 4,300 feet in 7 days. Process changes enabled a factory where 18 employees could not make enough parts for two Boeing 737-700s a month to produce parts for 23 aircraft a month with 14 employees.[1] Companies in a variety of other industries have made comparable improvements, often through data-driven management, process optimization, and technological acceleration.

Manufacturing companies are not alone in using such methods to boost productivity. WalMart achieved remarkable efficiency by optimizing management of the supply chain. Supermarkets used bar codes and scanners to accelerate checkout, improve customer service, manage inventories in real time, and reduce costs. Recently, supermarkets have used similar technologies for self-service checkout kiosks that reduce labor costs. Airport kiosks have enabled airlines to reduce passenger waiting times and labor requirements.

On the other hand, leading companies in some industries have been slow to recognize the effects of technological and market changes. Large, entrenched media companies, including companies that own newspapers, were for many years able to raise subscription prices and advertising rates as necessary to sustain business as usual. The big media companies were thus slow to understand how profoundly the internet would affect them. After waves of media mergers, many big media companies are still struggling.

The ability to raise prices as necessary to offset high costs has shielded drug companies from the need for greater efficiency in drug development. However, plentiful low-cost generics and a shift to considering cost along with efficacy in evaluating treatment options have recently undermined the industry's ability to increase prices at will. Furthermore, biotechnology companies and emerging competitors in developing countries are certain to intensify competition. The drug industry must respond to such sweeping changes.

The drug industry is already responding through downsizing and consolidation. However, reducing the number of competitors failed to protect big automotive and media companies. There is little reason to believe that such moves will reduce outside pressures for very different changes in the drug industry. On the contrary: downsizing and consolidation are likely to fuel demands for policies that dictate profound industry changes. A shrinking pool of competitors will add accusations of antitrust violations and price fixing to current complaints about high prices.

Health-care agencies, private insurers, businesses, and individual patients have reached a tipping point. They can no longer afford to meet the industry's price demands. Marginally superior drugs can no longer command markedly higher prices. Cost-effectiveness will increasingly decide whether hospitals, insurers, and agencies buy a product. There is no way around the central issue: to preserve its profits, and perhaps its independence, the drug industry must find a way to develop new products more efficiently.

Greater Efficiency: Changes That Everyone Can Applaud

Chapter 1 described a collection of forces that will increase the drug industry's challenges in decades to come, including: generic drugs; formularies; greater competition from biotechs and companies in emerging economies with low costs and growing scientific prowess; issues surrounding globalization and offshoring; the growing complexity of clinical studies; and individualized medicine. The barrier to addressing each of these challenges is high costs. Continued reliance on substantial price increases will not address these challenges but will intensify them. Stories about large price increases and disappointing results seem increasingly to go hand in hand.[2,3] Greater efficiency is the only way for the industry to address its major challenges.

The industry can best combat formularies and generics by introducing new drugs at prices proportional to improvements in efficacy over existing generics. The industry must learn to judge the cost-effectiveness of products in development and forecast pricing accordingly. In most therapeutic areas, the efficacy of low-cost generics will set the bar. Agile clinical development and its cornerstones, techniques for adapting study designs and operations, offer the most promising approach to competing successfully when the market standard is cost-effectiveness. Over time, techniques for adapting study designs promise to make clinical development a much more continuous process, reducing or eliminating between-phase delays. Besides reducing costs and shortening timelines, these techniques allow acquiring greater knowledge about test drugs earlier. Drugs that cost less to develop, reach market sooner, and appear in doses that provide maximum patient benefit will compete best on cost-effectiveness. Such drugs may allow the industry to maintain profits while moderating prices.

Operational adaptations can also help the industry meet the test of cost-effectiveness. Adaptive enrollment can exploit real-time data and performance metrics to reduce or eliminate delays in recruiting patient populations for studies as well as reducing costs by allocating recruitment funds to the most effective strategies. Adaptive monitoring can avoid the substantial waste that goes with allocating equal monitoring attention to all sites regardless of performance. Adaptive monitoring can also accelerate query resolution, promoting faster site closeout and database lock.

Many other aspects of agile development improve efficiency. For example, optimal data capture with electronic source documents—as provided by the digital pen and perhaps other technologies—greatly reduces the cost of source data verification. Lean processes combined with real-time data capture allow identifying and correcting the causes of queries early, reducing the number of queries in each study, the cost of query resolution, and the time required for database lock.

In summary, agile clinical development, incorporating both design and operational adaptations, offers the industry many ways to respond to the test of evaluation based on cost-effectiveness.

Biotechs and Emerging Low-Cost Competitors

Globalization and offshoring are accelerating the emergence of competitive drug companies in rapidly developing countries. These companies already provide intense competition by manufacturing low-cost generics. In time, the growing scientific prowess of these companies will combine with low costs to produce highly competitive novel drugs.

Despite the current credit crunch, biotechnology companies will, in the long term, continue to provide competition based on scientific leadership, specialization, and the advantage that smaller companies always enjoy—nimble response to changing circumstances. Inevitably, some of the researchers responsible for major scientific discoveries will form firms to create commercial products and wish to remain in control of their own fate. The drug industry cannot count on owning the most effective new drugs in every category, whether through internal development or acquisition.

In recent years, big pharma companies appear to have convinced themselves that they can reduce their own efforts in R&D, allowing smaller and more efficient companies to find winning drugs:

> The basic idea: Small biotech and pharma startups must prove the value of their ideas or perish from lack of funding. That often yields more promising candidates than internal research programs at a big pharma shop like Sanofi, where bureaucratic fiefdoms may keep unworthy ideas alive.[4]

With the winners identified at low cost, big drug companies expect to swoop down and purchase the most promising drug candidates. However, some candidates will not be for sale, and there is also some doubt about whether smaller companies are more efficient at drug development.[5] If not, reliance on outsourcing development may not reduce costs. Decisions to slash spending on R&D seem more calculated to meet short-term financial goals than to increase the output of new drugs or lower the cost of development. The attempt to become more efficient by acquiring the efficiency of others takes on an air of desperate rationalization.

Whether the industry develops new drugs in house or acquires them, greater competition will remain the reality. There will still in most cases be a struggle for acceptance in formularies, with some companies offering products at lower prices and other companies providing superior efficacy through innovative science. The industry's only safe response is to improve its own efficiency through design adaptations, operational adaptations, and other agile development techniques.

Although new competitors will sometimes have the advantage of lower costs or better science, they will also have disadvantages: limited resources and the need to establish themselves as legitimate alternatives to market leaders. Meticulous imitation of current industry development practices is the safest course for new competitors seeking acceptance in the marketplace and the medical community. This reality gives Big Pharma the opportunity to maintain an advantage by moving rapidly to agile clinical development even as new competitors mimic the inefficient methods that the drug industry is leaving behind.

Globalization, Offshoring, and Outsourcing

The drug industry has tried to reduce costs by offshoring work around the world. This has undeniably reduced the cost of certain development activities considered in isolation. However, great improvements in the efficiency of clinical development can come only from an integrated approach that optimizes development programs from start to finish. Efficient management of such integrated approaches demands the rapid flow of information to and from every unit involved. Reliance on antiquated batch processes impedes the flow of information and delays activities dependent on the work of distant contractors. Sending discrete activities offshore increases the challenge of integrating processes and maintaining an effective flow of information. Outside firms, regardless of location, must function as parts of an integrated whole. The industry must take care to ensure full integration and efficient communications.

Outsourcing, whether foreign or domestic, can make development more efficient provided drug companies view it strategically and integrate outsourced activities into an efficient development program. Such an approach to outsourcing makes outside service providers partners in development. Integration is not synonymous with ownership of all aspects of development and all companies involved. Henry Ford tried and failed to control the entire supply chain of materials for making cars—for example, from rubber plantations to tire plants to tires. As component suppliers became increasingly complex and specialized, this model evolved to one that inextricably linked the fate of assembler and supplier. Today, Toyota recognizes the interdependency by teaching suppliers how to increase efficiency and profits.[6]

The drug industry developed techniques for clinical research because they existed nowhere else. Later, the industry began to entrust CROs with minor studies and noncritical tasks. As CROs developed greater capabilities, sponsors increased efficiency and flexibility by turning to CROs not only for routine studies but also for challenging ones. To date, CROs have used the same conventional development methods as the industry. Contractors that use the same methods seem attractive to a risk-averse industry. However, because CROs relied on the same methods, they became commodity suppliers. The basis of competition was price, therapeutic specialization, and global reach. It was not the place of CROs to pioneer more efficient methods. Although CROs may sometimes achieve greater efficiency than their sponsors,[7] more efficient methods are not responsible for the improvement. In practice, many sponsors discourage or forbid their CRO suppliers from improving the sponsor's internal methods by formulating highly detailed specifications and permitting no deviations. Strategic relationships with CROs are rare; most sponsors discourage such thinking. Pharma sponsors manage contractors such as CROs tightly and at great expense to ensure compliance with internal company standards. The cost of managing a vendor, including identifying and selecting a vendor, negotiating and completing the contract, and overseeing work, is 10 times higher for pharmaceutical companies than for information technology vendors—4% versus 40%, respectively.[8]

In the current outsourcing model, sponsors focus largely on getting the greatest value for the dollar and CROs focus on assuring margins. The lack of common goals and incentives and long-term collaborative planning shows the tactical nature of the relationship. Other outsourcing arrangements are equally tactical. Wyeth's recent decision to outsource data management amounts to a strategy of offshoring to reduce costs rather than improve operational efficiency. Other large companies have either outsourced some portion of such activities or are exploring the possibility. Although the industry has always seen research as central to its mission, the industry has begun to outsource important research functions. Lilly has committed $1.6 billion to outsourcing portions of clinical research over the next decade.[9]

To make outsourcing a successful development strategy, drug companies and CROs must both develop new capabilities. Pharma companies must learn to integrate the work of outside suppliers into internal development processes without impeding workflow. CROs must provide services that readily integrate with drug company processes. Because CROs perform work for companies with different needs and processes, there is no simple formula for successful integration. To maximize efficiency, the agile development framework must evolve to help two companies function as one.

The framework of agile clinical development can address the challenge of integrating dispersed operations to maintain high efficiency. Computing and communications technology together with lean processes and active management based on real-time information can integrate and optimize development processes despite geographic dispersion, outsourcing, and offshoring. Outsourcing and offshoring are not an alternative to the agile approach to clinical development; rather, they make the adoption of the agile approach even more urgent.

Managing More Complex Trials

Clinical trials have become larger and more complex over time. There is every reason to expect this trend to continue. Larger patient populations and more complex protocols requiring more medical procedures have increased costs and stretched timelines. As noted above, geographic dispersion also complicates the management of clinical trials. Cost savings within specific outsourced operations do not necessarily reduce costs or shorten timelines for a development program taken as a whole. The challenge of managing across multiple organizations tends to cause delays, and longer timelines increase costs.

The industry can limit the cost of increased complexity by organizing work in integrated, lean processes and using technology to eliminate chokepoints. The industry must also learn to manage research through timely decision making based on real-time data, performance metrics, and performance analytics. By getting the right information to the right person at the right time, the industry can use distributed management to address complexity that could overwhelm a single decision maker atop a hierarchy. Efficient management based on real-time information, lean processes, and integrated systems is the best way to address the growing complexity of clinical studies.

Individualized Medicine Demands Greater Efficiency

Growing ability to define predictors of efficacy in individuals will usher in an era of personalized medicine. The transition to personalized medicine is well underway. Examples include routine testing of antibiotic sensitivity before treating infections and determining estrogen-receptor status before prescribing chemotherapy for breast cancer. In the future, thousands of individual markers will guide medical decisions by predicting some aspect of response to different treatments. Handheld devices for instant, complete, individualized diagnosis exist only in science fiction. However, science has taken the first steps in that direction.

Improved prediction of efficacy and safety will change the administration of screening programs. Large-scale screening programs for prostate, breast, and colon cancer already modify general guidelines for specific risk factors. Both diagnosis and treatment will rely increasingly on individual risk markers. For example, screening guidelines differ for women known to have genetic markers such as *BrCa1* and *BrCa2*. Large-scale cost-benefit analyses suggest directing more expensive tests such as breast CT scans to patients at greatest risk.

Cancer immunotherapy will be among the fields that lead the way to individualized therapy. More than 100 single-nucleoside polymorphisms (SNPs) identify DNA variations that influence risk of common human diseases. Predictive algorithms must consider not only the collective effect of such individual markers but also such other factors as the degree to which genetic differences are expressed (proteinomics) and environmental and dietary influences. Growing knowledge and refinement of techniques for analyzing multiple markers and risk factors will inevitably increase the precision of diagnosis and treatment choices, accelerating the transition to individualized medicine. The immune system offers such potential for treating even widespread cancer that an editorial in the *New England Journal of Medicine* has proclaimed the "beginning of the endgame"—the goal of harnessing the patient's own immune system to repulse cells that have begun to multiply uncontrollably.[10]

It is no longer farfetched to imagine a world in which individualized screening programs identify diseases much earlier than is currently possible. Testing of cancerous cells following diagnosis will resemble current sensitivity testing on any new infection. Individual characteristics will drive the formulation of specific drugs to address the needs of each patient.

The increasing individualization of medicine has profound implications for drug development methods. Rather than testing new treatments on many thousands of people with unknown differences, researchers will have to test new drugs on smaller, targeted populations, perhaps only hundreds or even tens of individuals. Large populations allow statistical adjustments for some characteristics that affect outcome. For example, gender, age, and cholesterol levels influence the development and progression of heart disease. In small samples defined by factors such as individual genetic markers, controlling for such characteristics will be far more difficult. Smaller samples will also greatly reduce the ability to adjust for different background risk by stratification or restriction, the two statistical methods currently used. Furthermore, small samples make achieving significant *p*-values difficult even when the treatment effect is strong.

Individualized medicine also has profound implications for the economics of drug development. Genetically targeted medicines inherently address smaller markets. To serve small markets profitably, the industry must find more efficient approaches to development. Although genetic testing itself imposes high costs, current inefficient development practices present an even greater problem. The industry cannot spend $1.2 billion to develop each drug for a market far too small to generate commensurate revenues and profits. The principles of agile clinical research and its cornerstones, design adaptations and operational adaptations, can help by greatly reducing overall development timelines and costs.

A More Important Role for Postmarketing Studies

The shift from large-scale studies of drugs for large target populations will likely limit the amount of information collected before approval of new drugs. The approval process already presents formidable challenges for both developers and regulators. However, smaller study populations for targeted treatments may force decisions about approving promising new treatments based on the response of fewer people. Closer postapproval scrutiny will be essential as more people use new products in a greater variety of real-world situations, including unanticipated concurrent use with other products. The need to look for infrequent events will also mandate new methods.

Data based on smaller samples exacerbates a dilemma that regulators have long confronted—that of approving a product for marketing and allowing physicians to prescribe for any use they see fit, including "off-label" conditions. One strategy for addressing this issue would be graduated introduction of new drugs. Increasing experience and reassurance about safety and efficacy would justify expanded availability of the new drug.

Researchers may have to take greater responsibility for providing oversight after products reach market. Postmarketing studies to date are generally limited in number and scope. Regulators are demanding more attention to postmarketing studies, mostly to better define safety. The need for more information increases the already high costs of drug development. However, the technologies and processes described in this book can reduce the cost of collecting postmarketing data. Compared to the cost of recognizing safety issues years after a drug reaches market, efficient postmarketing studies may serve as cost-effective tripwires. Postmarketing studies can also provide a cost-effective means of assessing the performance of a product in real-world settings and specific subpopulations. What is required is a large-scale, inexpensive means of casting a wide net for new information combined with determination to dig deeper when indicated. Current technology can support this approach. Electronic medical records will further reduce the costs of postmarketing studies.

The ability to identify areas of interest at low cost and look more closely at areas of concern can have enormous value. Perhaps the clearest illustration of the value of this approach is in large-scale cohort studies such as Harvard's Physician Health Study and Nurses' Health Study. Both followed large groups of health professionals over time. Subjects completed follow-up questionnaires at regular intervals. However, the studies could also issue more detailed follow-up questionnaires for any emerging issues of concern.

Postmarketing studies offer additional value by allowing detailed product comparisons. Many companies see postmarketing efforts as "bad news only" studies that identify and publicize safety issues. However, besides limiting the repercussions of safety issues, postmarketing studies can provide information on positive attributes that allow greater product differentiation. Taking advantage of this possibility requires efficient integrated processes for collecting and analyzing information. The same integrated, technology-driven approach that improves the efficiency of preapproval studies can optimize postmarketing studies.

The Reward for Greater Efficiency

Chapter 6 described cost and time savings from the use of the agile approach, including design and operational adaptations, throughout a hypothetical development program. Figure 10-1 contrasts the timelines for the same program conducted with traditional methods and the agile approach.

The direct time and cost savings from agile clinical development can be great. The indirect effect on the value of investments can be greater still. The agile approach reduces the time required for conducting each phase, the time between studies, and the time required for regulatory filings. Chapter 6 described how the agile approach could shorten a specific, hypothetical development program from about seven years to less than four, a reduction of 58%.

These timelines may strike researchers accustomed to conventional methods as implausible. Certainly, there is an enormous gulf between today's norm and the timelines shown. However, combined and comprehensive use of the techniques described in this book can achieve results that are implausible with conventional methods. Widespread acceptance of today's typical performance provides no evidence to refute the claim that the agile approach can greatly shorten timelines and reduce costs. Dramatic improvements are not only plausible, but also attainable and necessary.

When a top-priority General Motors program needed seven years to develop a new sedan, Honda was able to develop a new Accord in four.[11] A study found that developing a new Japanese car from first design to customer deliveries took on average 46 months and 1,700,000 engineering hours. The average United States and European models took 60 months and 3,000,000 engineering hours.[6] Achieving better results in less time with less effort and lower costs shows what huge improvements companies can make when determined to improve and willing to change existing development processes. For the drug industry, the first step to more efficient development is realizing that large improvements are possible. The industry must view today's typical performance at drug development as a compelling reason to embrace adaptive methods and agile clinical development quickly and comprehensively.

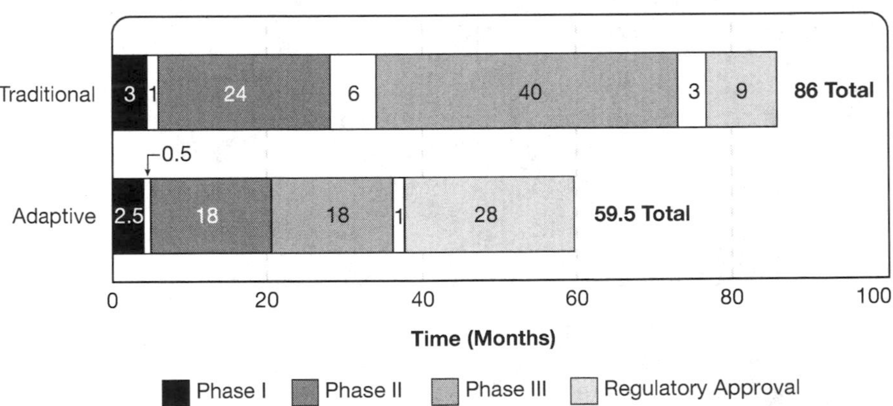

Figure 10-1. Comparison of traditional and fully adaptive study timelines. This assumes a baseline study that might take about seven years from beginning to submission of regulatory application. The numbers below each segment indicate duration in months. Adaptive techniques enable reducing each phase and reducing or eliminating between-study gaps. (This example is intended to show typical results; time savings in each program depend on individual study circumstances and characteristics.) White indicates between-phase study pauses. Progressively lighter shades of gray indicate traditional development phases I, II, and III. The lightest shade represents regulatory approval time.

Source: Health Decisions, Inc. Used by permission.

Table 10-1 summarizes the scale of the savings by phase and adaptive or agile technique.

Table 10-1. Typical savings in time and cost and the range of savings possible through agile development programs.

	Operational	Design	Typical	Range
Safety testing	Rapid decision cycles	CRM*	35%	15–80%
Dose finding	Rapid enrollment	SSRE§	25%	10–35%
	Centralized monitoring	Adaptive randomization		
	Reduced rework	Pruning		
	Rapid database lock	Seamless transition		
Confirmatory	Rapid enrollment	SSRE§	30%	10–25%
	Centralized monitoring	Pruning		
	Reduced rework			
	Rapid database lock			
Regulatory Submission	Earlier start on preparation based on indication of success		20%	10–40%

*Continuous reassessment method

§SSRE=Sample size reestimation

Note: Percentage savings in time and cost are similar. While some studies and programs will be unable to take advantage of some techniques, these figures estimate typical improvements. These figures exclude potentially substantial savings from eliminating delays between phases.

Financial Implications of the Agile Approach

The financial consequences of the agile approach for an entire development program are more striking than the cost savings for each component phase. Two financial measures for evaluating investments show how time savings improve investment prospects. Internal rate of return (IRR) gauges the efficiency or quality of an investment. The IRR estimates the annualized rate of growth that the investment is expected to produce on the initial investment—the investment's yield. An IRR higher than the cost of capital yields a profit. A substantial IRR on a large investment will pay off handsomely; even a great IRR on a tiny investment will produce limited gains in absolute terms.

Net present value (NPV) estimates the size of the gain that an investment will produce. The NPV is the difference between the expected future cash flows from an investment and the amount of the investment. NPV compares the value of an investment to the rate of return that the same amount of money would earn if invested with similar risks in financial markets. NPV discounts the value of future cash flows to equivalent dollar amounts at the time of the analysis. Any prospective investment with a positive NPV, an excess of cash flows, will produce a gain. Any prospective investment with a negative NPV, a shortfall of cash flows, will produce a loss. If an investment is large enough, a drug could make a large profit despite having a low IRR. However, investing the same amount of money in a drug with a substantially higher IRR would make much more money. In investment decisions, drug companies are seeking both a high percentage gain and a large absolute gain—both a high IRR and a large NPV.

Development times profoundly affect IRR and NPV. Suppose a company expects a new drug to reach modest peak annual sales of $300 million and the drug takes six years to develop with conventional methods. Based on traditional assumptions about tax rate, discount rate, and cost of capital, such a product would have an NPV of $280 million. The program would produce an IRR of 65%. Both these measures of investment prospects signal a product worthy of investment.

It would be reasonable to expect agile techniques to shorten the timelines and reduce costs for phase I by 25% and to reduce the gap between this first stage and subsequent stages by one-third. Using a full-fledged agile approach for phase II, the reduction in timeline and cost would likely be 40% and the reduction in the gap would be one-quarter; for phase III, reductions in timeline and costs would be 35% and 8%, respectively. With full use of agile methods from the outset, the total reduction in timeline and cost would likely be 35% over a conventional approach, with a range of 10%–50%. Such savings would increase the NPV to $636 million and the IRR to 144%. These numbers represent a 128% increase in NPV and 115% improvement in IRR.

For larger projects, the agile approach produces similar benefits. However, the absolute number of dollars is strikingly higher. Recall that the discontinued torcetrapib development program had costs estimated at $800 million.[12] Developing drugs of this class frequently costs more because the target audience is so large. Studies use large samples to gather more extensive information than usual before exposing a potentially huge population. In the case of torcetrapib, the confirmatory study included 15,000 patients. With such a large development program, even a modest application of agile methods could save substantial time and money. Phase II testing would consume on the order of 35% of total costs for a program on this scale, or about $280 million. Using the agile approach for phase II in such a program could reduce timelines by several years and costs by approximately $70 million.

The full-scale application of agile methods in all phases of a medium-sized or large program would likely increase the NPV by 100% (Figure 10-2), with corresponding increases in IRR. The absolute savings in phase I might be modest compared to savings from larger and more expensive late-stage studies. However, time saved in phase I would still greatly improve the outlook for the investment by reducing time to market. For a development program with $75 million budget and expected peak annual sales of $500 million, application of agile techniques to shorten phase I would increase the NPV by $71 million and increase the IRR 4%.

Figure 10-2 shows the increases in NPV likely in each of three phases as development costs increase. These figures are consistent with estimates of the effects of shortening development times developed by DiMasi.[13] Figures presented in this book suggest that DiMasi's estimates may be conservative because those estimates considered reductions in capitalized costs though shortening development time. Agile development can not only shorten timelines but also reduce the direct cost of developing pharmaceutical products.

Since development programs vary widely, a single example may be less instructive than exploring the effects of different development assumptions with an interactive calculator. One such calculator is available online (www.healthdec.com/adaptive). The calculator allows gauging the estimated impact of using the agile approach in any of the three phases separately or in combination. Users can vary expected peak sales as well as cost and duration of development. While the specific effects of agile clinical development will vary, most programs are likely to realize substantial savings in costs and timelines and substantial improvements in NPV and IRR.

To be sure, it is unreasonable to expect every program to achieve all of the improvements described in the hypothetical development program in Chapter 6. It will not always be possible to move seamlessly from safety to dose finding and to move seamlessly again from dose finding to confirmatory studies. In other cases, savings from SSRE may be less than those in the hypothetical program, or savings from adaptive enrollment or adaptive monitoring may be less. Nevertheless, comprehensive use of the agile approach throughout most programs can reduce timelines substantially. Achieving half the time savings from the example in Chaper 6 would substantially improve financial indicators.

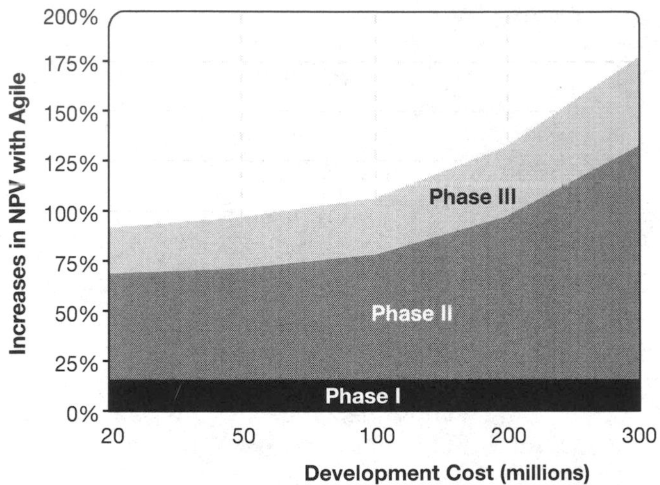

Figure 10-2. Improvements in efficiency and NPV from agile clinical development, by phase and development program cost, where cost is based on conventional development. Savings are greatest in phase II, especially as program size and complexity increase.

Financial Implications of the Agile Approach for the Drug Industry

If the agile approach can provide substantial benefits for clinical studies and great benefits for development programs, the benefits for the drug industry as a whole can be enormous. Recall that PhRMA members reported investing approximately $44 billion in R&D in 2007. Recall also that clinical research accounts for 70% of the $403 million in average out-of-pocket costs and 64% of average development time of 11.8 years for each new drug.[14] Based on these figures, assume that clinical development costs represent 60% of the annual investment by PhRMA members in R&D. In any year, parts of the industry's R&D spending go to products in every stage of clinical development. However, the distribution of investment among early, middle, and late development activities is reasonably consistent from year to year, with larger late-stage studies consuming more of the investment and smaller early-stage studies less. For simplicity, assume that the industry is spending $44 billion on R&D in a specific year on new projects expected to mature after approximately 10 years and that $26 billion of this is spent on clinical development. What sort of an effect would an industry-wide switch to the agile approach have on the NPV of such a $26 billion annual investment as against continued use of the current approach?

If we assume that the savings in cost and time from using the agile approach for all the industry's clinical development activities would be proportional to the benefits shown in the hypothetical development program described in Chapter 6 and summarized here (roughly 20% cost savings, 50% time savings), the net savings would be approximately $5 billion and just under three years of development time. The new generation of products starting in the clinical pipeline in 2010 would mature in 2015 instead of 2017. The cost of clinical development would be $39 billion instead of $44 billion. The NPV of products with $26 billion in annual clinical spending in 2010 would be on the order of $208 billion* rather than $111 billion with the current approach (Figure 10-3). With even half of the savings noted above, the same assumptions increase the NPV from $111 billion under a traditional approach to $161 billion.

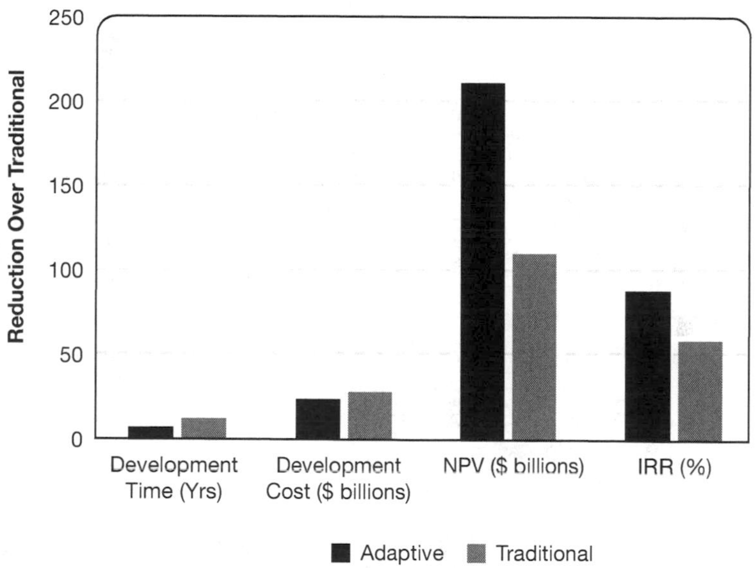

Figure 10-3. In broad strokes based on simplifying assumptions, the effect of the agile approach to clinical development on the NPV of the drug industry's aggregate annual spending on clinical R&D compared to the conventional approach.

* Based on sales life of 15 years that includes development time and peak sales of 6 times development cost. This number is an approximation because expenditures in any year include products at various stages of development, while, for simplicity, this example assumes all products are at the same stage.

A Brighter Future for Clinical Development

The potential gains from applying adaptive concepts to the design and operational aspects of clinical development are too powerful to pass up. Agile clinical development—the approach described in this book—stands ready to pave the way to a brighter future for a drug industry currently beset by unprecedented challenges. The agile approach can shift the primary strategic focus from retrenchment to product development—long the lifeblood of the pharmaceutical industry. Future success for the drug industry lies in developing greater numbers of compelling new products more rapidly and at lower cost. Agile clinical development can help the industry achieve this goal. Now is the time to begin the transition to the agile approach.

First Steps toward Agile Development

Whether the credit for improvements in the processes of clinical research goes to lean thinking, Peter Drucker's mandate to give managers information to manage by, or other management approaches such as reengineering business processes, the core idea is the same: Conduct more efficient studies by optimizing processes and making timely decisions based on current information. Debate about applying any one management approach and, in particular, debate about whether lean thinking is appropriate in clinical research should not distract the industry's focus from these key points:

- The best way to achieve the necessary improvement in the efficiency of clinical development is to adopt a more vigorous and responsive approach to management characterized by midcourse decision making using current study information.
- Since study designs do not account for all the inefficiency in clinical research, adapting study designs cannot fix the entire problem.
- Management based on current study information should seek to optimize not only study designs but also study operations.

Lean thinking is no doubt among the useful ways of examining the efficiency and quality of work processes to identify and eliminate waste, optimize resource allocation, minimize rework, and so on. However, in the author's view, adopting all aspects of the lean approach is probably overkill in clinical development, at least for the present. Many critical processes in clinical development remain strikingly inefficient. Nuances of management doctrine matter less at this stage than a focus on the use of current study information to stamp out the most glaring inefficiencies. There can be enormous gains in efficiency simply from conducting studies based on rapid data collection and validation, continuous generation of performance metrics and analytics on study operations, careful use of established methods of adapting study designs, and decision making as necessary to optimize the course of each study.

Thus, agile clinical development, with adaptive research at its core, gives the drug industry an alternative to seeking salvation primarily through the elimination of people and programs and increased reliance on offshoring. The industry can also take advantage of readily available techniques to make R&D much more efficient. These techniques can yield substantial improvements regardless of where studies take place and whether pharma company staff or outside contractors conduct the studies. The gains in efficiency can simultaneously reduce the cost of drug development and increase the output of new drugs, generating additional revenues by satisfying market demands.

The scale of waste in clinical development is likely on the order of the 25–40% estimated for the health-care system as a whole[15] and for drug manufacturing.[16] Therefore, the savings from the application of a more vigorous and data-driven management approach can be enormous—great enough to constitute a major new source of funding for drug development. Furthermore, the savings can make potential markets profitable that now seem too small for pharma development to address. With savings from greater efficiencies in clinical research, the drug industry will be able to make profits on personalized medicines and niche markets such as those now addressed by "orphan" drugs. Reduced development costs will also allow maintaining profits on medicines with wider clinical applications without such heavy reliance on price increases. Over time, this can reduce public and political pressures on the industry.

For all these reasons, the industry should move rapidly to embrace agile clinical development. This means taking concrete steps (see below). The ability to adapt study designs using sophisticated new techniques deserves consideration in planning each and every study. The industry should mandate the use of real-time information to adapt study operations in all clinical studies. The combined use of design and operational adaptations can not only improve the industry's efficiency but also enable the industry to profit from the dawning era of individualized medicine and to increase its output of new products of all types. Organizing work in lean processes, making timely decisions based on real-time information, and using distributed management techniques can all provide substantial improvements in clinical development programs. As a result, the industry will be able to improve the treatment of the numerous health conditions that afflict hundreds of millions of people all over the world. In time, public outcries against drug prices may give way to some measure of gratitude for the fruits of drug industry research.

An Eight-Point Program for Embracing the Adaptive Approach

- Put an adaptive platform in place (Chapter 9).
- Start design adaptations with small steps, such as CRM in dose finding and other early adaptations.
- Consider sample-size reestimation for each study with expected sample size greater than 100.
- Begin the use of operational adaptations with adaptive enrollment.
- Expand to adaptive monitoring.
- Start using electronic source documents with data-capture technologies such as the digital pen, revolutionizing source data verification.
- Move to combined phase studies, combining safety testing with efficacy, and phase IIb dose-selection studies with phase III confirmatory trials.
- Optimize the combined use of design and operational adaptations to achieve agile development.

References

1 Pollack P. Aerospace gets Japan's message; without military largess, industry takes the lean path. New York Times. Mar 9, 1999.

2 Martinez B, Johnson A. Drug makers, hospitals raise prices. Wall Street J. Apr 15, 2009.

3 Loftus, P. US drug market faces down year. Wall Street J. Apr 23, 2009.

4 Goldstein J. Sanofi-Aventis CEO looks to cut research spending. Wall Street J Health Blog. Mar 6, 2009. Available from: http://blogs.wsj.com/health/2009/03/06/sanofi-aventis-ceo-looks-to-cut-research-spending/.

5 Pisano GP. Science Business. Boston: Harvard Business School Press; 2006.

6 Womack J, Jones D. Lean thinking. 1st Free Press Edition. New York: Simon & Schuster; 2003. p. 69.

7 Kaitin KI, editor. CRO contribution to drug development is substantial and growing globally. Tufts Center for the Study of Drug Development Impact Report 2006 Jan/Feb;8(1).

8 Anderson B. How we fail to use CROs effectively. Applied Clin Trials. 2008;8:42–8.

9 Christel M. Long-term investment. R&D Directions. 2008;14:20–7.

10 Weiner LM. Focus on research: cancer immunotherapy: the endgame begins. N Engl J Med. 2008;358:2664–5.

11 Womack J, Jones D, Roos D. The machine that changed the world. First HarperPerennial Edition. New York: HarperCollins; 1991. pp. 109–10.

12 Winslow R. After Pfizer blockbuster's failure, what's next for the heart? Wall Street J. Dec 5, 2006.

13 DiMasi J. The value of improving the productivity of the drug development process. Pharmacoeconomics. 2002;20:Suppl 3:1–10.

14 DiMasi J, Hansen R, Grabowski H. The price of innovation: new estimates of drug development costs. J Health Econ. 2003;22:151–85.

15 Scanlon J, Berwick D. Curing the healthcare system. How Dr. Donald Berwick and the Institute for Healthcare Improvement apply business best practices—from lean manufacturing to innovation. Business Week. Nov 17, 2008. Available from: http://www.businessweek.com/innovate/content/nov2008/id20081117_820750_page_2.htm.

16 Improvement tip: find muda and root it out. Institute for Healthcare Improvement. Cambridge MA. Oct 2005;53. Accessed Dec 27, 2008. Available from: http://www.ihi.org/IHI/Topics/Improvement/ImprovementMethods/ImprovementStories/ImprovementTipFindMudaandRootitOut.htm.

Index